To Sammull & Michael:

It's a privilege being your eye Doctor.

Dr. D.

A PARENT'S GUIDE TO
RAISING CHILDREN WITH
HEALTHY VISION

This book is intended to be informational and should not be considered a substitute for advice from an eye doctor, whom the reader should consult before undertaking any of the suggestions within this book. The parents and children featured in this book are actual patients who were not paid for their stories. Their results may or may not be indicative of your child's treatment. Treatments to control myopia are not suitable for every patient and are not risk free. The information in this book is for general knowledge only.

The authors and publisher expressly disclaim responsibility for any adverse effects arising from the use or application of the information contained in this book.

FIRST EDITION

Designed by Meridith Feldman, Skylographic Design

ISBN: 978-0-692-11394-3

Note from authors: *Throughout the book we've referred to eye professionals as "eye doctors." There is understandably confusion among patients, since there is more than one type of provider of vision care and not all of them are doctors. Most likely your child's vision care will involve optometrists, opticians and ophthalmologists.*

Each plays an important and unique role in maintaining a child's clear and healthy vision. We recommend working with the eye professional who treats your child (and you) with respect in a competent and comprehensive manner. Let your instinct be your guide, not the eye professional's degree, insurance plan participation or their office location. In our office we are privileged to work with all three types of eye professionals, since each fulfills specific needs for our patients.

Thank you to Meridith Feldman, Paragon Vision Sciences, Shutterstock, and Theodore Kaye for their photographs.

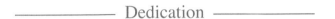 Dedication

To my parents, Vasilios and Allegra
For enduring so much to afford their
children a healthier life

Nicholas Despotidis

To my parents, Barry and Sandi
For their unconditional love and support

Noah Tannen

Acknowledgments

Blaise Pascal, the French mathematician, is attributed with saying, "I have only made this letter longer because I have not had the time to make it shorter." The succinctness of this manuscript, outlining a very complex health issue, is a result of the sum total of those who gave of themselves to actualize this book. First and foremost, to my co-author Noah Tannen; your ability to write with ease and your commitment to accuracy is an inspiration. To Kimberly Lee, who undertook the task of writing her chapter and sharing her family's personal challenges for the sheer purpose of helping other parents, thank you for your words.

To our editors from Wink Productions, your encouragement and professionalism was instrumental in articulating our thoughts accurately and succinctly. To Meridith Feldman, who designed the cover and entire book, your talents are multidimensional. To Michele Horner, thank you for undertaking the tedious task of editing the initial manuscript and helping it come to life. To my good friend and confidant, Howard Feldman, thank you for providing unconditional support...always with a critical eye. To Jamie Sussel Turner, M. Ed., you epitomize what it means to be a great coach. To Richard Jeffries, president of Paragon Vision Sciences, your success mirrors the value you provide to others. Thank you to Maria Liu, OD, PhD, for having the fortitude and conviction to pioneer the first clinic devoted to myopia control, and for your insight in the development of this manuscript. Thank you to Craig Norman for continually supporting my projects by providing valuable insight. And thank you to Kurtis Schmidt for his help at every stage of this book's development.

To our professional reviewers, your insights were invaluable: Jay Hochheiser, LCSW; Aimee Goodman, DO; Shunli Hou, MD; Steve Jacobs, OD; Leah Johnson, OD; Bruce Koffler, MD; Paul Levine, OD; Michael Lipson, OD; Eef van der Worp, BOptom, PhD.

To Jay Zenker, your suggestions made our message more cohesive and comprehensible, thank you!

To the parents who cared enough to review and provide feedback: James Bash, Mike Graff, Jamie Huang-Teng, Angela Kneppers, Jennifer Mullen, Eileen Porada, and Mona Young.

To all the families who allowed us to use their family photos in our book, I'm so proud to have included you: the Bash, Brown, Kneppers, Kushner, Morshed, and Shafer families.

Thank you to our office manager, Lisa M. MacArthur, who rules with a big stick and an even bigger heart; and to our technician, Laurel Whitehead, for her commitment to detail. To our entire staff, without you we're just an ordinary medical office.

But most all, to my wife, Teresa, and our children, Nicholas and Gregory, who inspired this book.

Foreword

When I first met Dr. Despotidis, we immediately connected; simply because we share the same philosophy about how to treat nearsightedness in children. Rather than manage a condition (myopia), we look beyond the child's vision. Instead of offering a temporary treatment, we are providing lifelong guidance about lifestyle and visual habits. Aside from being eye doctors, we are their friends, teachers, and counselors.

As the founder of the first myopia control clinic in an academic setting, I have encountered plenty of resistance. My attempts to implement evidence-based research into a clinical setting were often met with skepticism from inside and outside our profession. I cannot imagine how much Dr. Despotidis encountered as he began his focus on controlling myopia among children over a decade earlier.

Why are we so passionate in the face of such resistance? The answer lies in those moments when we witness children light up upon seeing clearly for the first time without their eyeglasses. Our resolve is strengthened when students return for their check-ups and tell us how much better they perform at school and in sports without eyeglasses! It is when the child engages in conversation with us, but is now using direct eye contact, exuding strong confidence. These priceless moments make it clear, as these children's eye doctors, we're not just managing their myopia--we're helping transform them into happier, more confident, more socially amicable people.

A Parent's Guide to Raising Children with Healthy Vision offers cutting-edge knowledge and recommendations in a highly objective manner, while remaining surprisingly easy to read and understand. I can say with great certainty that the authors will acquire many appreciative parents who can relate to the stories and suggestions in this book, and who will gain a much broader and deeper perspective of what it entails to nurture happy children with healthy vision.

Yue (Maria) Liu, OD, PhD, MPH, MBA, FAAO
Assistant Professor of Clinical Optometry
Chief of Myopia Control Clinic
University of California, Berkeley

Contents

Introduction

In 2009 I co-wrote a book in response to the growing number of children wearing eyeglasses to correct myopia or nearsightedness titled *My Children Are Nearsighted Too*. Since that time, the number of children wearing eyeglasses to correct myopia has continued to grow at an alarming rate. We are currently in the midst of what researchers refer to as "the myopia epidemic."[1] According to the U.S. National Health and Nutrition Examination Survey, rates of myopia in the United States have increased 66% since 1971.[2] In many East Asian countries, myopia incidence rates have climbed as high as 80 to 90% among adolescents.[2] If something is not done now to curb this trend, researchers project that one half of the world's population (in other words, 5 billion people) will be myopic by the year 2050![3]

What's happening to our children and their eyesight? The answer to this question is outlined in the book you are holding in your hands, *A Parent's Guide to Raising Children with Healthy Vision*. I've gathered my insight after 30 years of examining and treating children for visual problems. As a doctor, I've spoken to thousands of parents who share one common goal: to raise healthy children in every sense of the word... physically, emotionally, and socially. This book is written to educate parents on the science behind myopia development and the serious consequences technology has on our children's social development.

I wrote *My Children Are Nearsighted Too* as a father who happens to be an eye doctor, feeling helpless as I witnessed my two sons' eyesight deteriorate. *A Parent's Guide to Raising Children with Healthy Vision* continues that journey along with my sons, both of whom have graduated from college and entered adulthood.

To provide a balanced perspective, I've enlisted the help of my younger colleague, Noah Tannen, and Kimberly Lee, a teacher with a Master in Education. Each brings a different viewpoint to raising children with healthy vision. Kim shares her insight as a mother of three and a teacher with an advanced degree in counseling psychology. I've known Kim for over two decades; her ability to see the forest when it comes to child development is extraordinary and I'm very excited she has shared her wisdom in this multi-factorial dilemma of childhood vision deterioration.

Dr. Noah Tannen is a young colleague who has yet to start a family. I co-wrote my first book with his father, Barry Tannen. "Dr. Noah," as his patients call him, provides insight from someone who had access to a computer as a child, uses and enjoys social media, yet has profound respect for the impact it has on eyesight. He's completed a residency in pediatric vision and vision rehabilitation, and has spoken extensively on the topic of myopia development, stabilization, and avenues for possible prevention. Most importantly, he empathizes with our younger patients whose lives revolve around mobile technology. Interestingly, Dr. Noah never developed nearsightedness, despite years of electronic and academic rigors. He'll discuss his insight into this as well.

Life is not black and white; there is no formula for raising healthy, happy children. Every child is unique. That's the power of this book. It's filled with facts, insights, and recommendations, but ultimately it's a tool to allow parents to make the best decisions for their own children when it comes to vision. My hope is for parents to see the world through our eyes; as eye doctors, parents, and advocates for non-conformity.

—Nick Despotidis, OD, FAAO, FCOVD, FIAOMC

The Epidemic

Nicholas Despotidis

*Myopia is predicted to affect
1 in every 2 people by the year 2050.
It plagues our children and it has no cure.*[3]

My wife and I were excited, but nervous, as we drove to the mall to pick up the family portraits we had taken the month before. Twenty years ago, long before the advent of digital cameras, it was our tradition to gather our sons, slick down their hair, and drive to the portrait studio to capture a memory in our family's timeline. While we were always eager for this event, we were always just a little bit anxious, too.

"Were the boys' eyes open?"
"Were their smiles natural?"
*"What if there was a wardrobe malfunction
that we had missed?"*

As the envelope containing our pictures was opened, my wife and I beamed with joy! Our boys, Nicholas, 9, and Gregory, 6, looked great! Their green and blue plaid shirts enhanced their beautiful eyes and their smiles were heartwarming. What a relief!

But as I stared at the 8 x 11 matted portrait, my attention was drawn to their eyeglasses. I had forgotten that Nicholas and Gregory wore their glasses during the photoshoot because they wore them all the

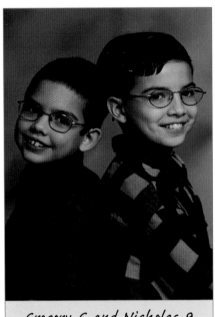

Gregory, 6, and Nicholas, 9

time. I had been practicing optometry for over a decade when that portrait was taken. Prescribing glasses was my *job*; it consumed the majority of my day. Yet, as a father, I was dismayed when I saw my young sons wearing their glasses in the family portrait. Of course they looked cute, these distinguished, bespectacled young men, but at that very moment, my professional life changed.

I had learned in optometry school that kids wore glasses because their parents passed along a gene that contributed to their poor eyesight. However, my wife and I didn't start wearing glasses until much later in life. Why were my sons wearing glasses at such a young age?

Long before seeing that family portrait, I knew there was a major flaw in that theory. At the beginning of my career as an eye doctor, the incidence of myopia among children in the United States was approximately 25%.[2] Yet, I felt as if I was prescribing more and more eyeglasses for nearsighted children every year. Maybe it was because children having trouble seeing the chalkboard were the ones who sought my care? After all, children who passed the vision screening in the school nurse's office would not need my help. But, that belief unraveled as my sons' eyesight continued to deteriorate throughout elementary school.

In my first book, *My Children Are Nearsighted Too*, I delved into the possibility that lifestyle also affects children's eyesight. I addressed commonly asked questions:

Does TV negatively impact children's eyesight?
What about reading in poor light?
Does bad posture affect eyesight?
Do computer games play a role in deteriorating vision?

There is no doubt in my mind, ALL of the above situations affect a child's vision, and my book outlined research demonstrating environmental factors that play a significant role in the development of nearsightedness in kids. My coauthors and I also outlined some of the treatments available to parents who consider alternative vision correction for their children. Some of these treatments are even shown to slow down the progression of myopia.

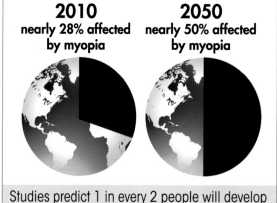

2010
nearly 28% affected
by myopia

2050
nearly 50% affected
by myopia

Studies predict 1 in every 2 people will develop myopia by the year 2050, a projected 5 BILLION people.[3]

Myopia continues to increase at an alarming rate. Studies comparing the incidence of myopia in the United States from 1971 to 2004 document a 66% increase.[2] The rise among children needing eyeglasses is even more disturbing in many East Asian countries. The prevalence in some parts of China and Taiwan are reported as high as 90%. In Korea, almost 96% of college students require eyeglasses to correct for myopia.[1] The World Health Organization considers myopia among children to be approaching epidemic proportions.[4]

> Myopia continues to increase at an alarming rate.

When I began practicing optometry, most parents were concerned that poor vision was impacting their child's baseball swing, not their school grades. Today in my practice, it seems that extracurricular activities have been sidelined by the rigors of school and homework.

What is Going On?

Clearly, something is going on, but researchers can't agree on exactly what that something is. Animal studies support the theory that experiencing a blurred image on the retina at the back of the eye can induce myopia.[5] Other studies highlight the fact that children spend less time playing outdoors, especially in countries with conveniences such as computers, smartphones, air-conditioning, and televisions. Can it simply be lack of sunlight causing this alarming spike in children wearing eyeglasses?

> The World Health Organization considers myopia among children to be approaching epidemic proportions.

My clinical intuition leads me to believe there are multiple factors contributing to the myopia epidemic including a genetic predisposition, the amount of time a child spends indoors, as well as the intensity with which a student concentrates on near work. And in my opinion, the degree of scholastic competition to which children are exposed also likely plays a role.

And there is one more possible factor in the myopia epidemic: electronics.

"It's too hot outside!"
"It's too cold to go outside!"
*"There is no one to play with me outside, that's why
I stay inside after school."*

The excuses are many and kids don't have to go outside to be entertained. As a matter of fact, many would rather entertain themselves on their screens than play outside.

What is Myopia?

Simply stated, myopia is a disease. Myopia is a visual condition where a person cannot see clearly at a distance, but sees clearly up close. This is why it is commonly referred to as "nearsightedness" or "shortsightedness." In this book, we interchange the terms "nearsightedness" and "myopia."

Myopia can be inherited. If one parent wears eyeglasses to correct nearsightedness, their child has approximately a 20% chance of also needing eyeglasses. If both parents are nearsighted, the probability of their offspring developing myopia more than doubles![6]

In my office, more and more children require eyeglasses to correct nearsightedness. That's a fact.[7]

Why the Fuss about Myopia?

Most parents seek my care because of their child's increasing dependence on eyewear. But this condition is more than an inconvenience. There are long term consequences associated with myopia. Glasses, contact lenses, and surgery will improve vision, but they do not address the underlying issue; the higher the degree of myopia, the more elongated the eyeball becomes. This elongation of the eye stretches and thins out the inner parts of the eye (retina), which increases the risk of several side effects. Some sight-threatening conditions commonly associated with myopia are:[8]

- retinal detachment
- cataracts
- glaucoma
- macular degeneration

AN OUNCE OF PREVENTION IS WORTH A POUND OF CURE
AS TOLD BY DR. D

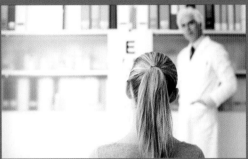

Doctors can experience sight threatening side effects of myopia, too

I recall being riveted to my seat while the world renowned researcher spoke on the topic of myopia. He warned the doctors in attendance about the growing levels of high myopia that are increasing the risks of serious eye conditions, which may lead to permanent blindness. You could hear a pin drop in the auditorium. Most of us viewed myopia as an inconvenience, correctable with eyeglasses or contacts, but a risk for permanent blindness? Up until that moment, I did not connect the increasing prevalence of myopia with the associated increased risk of side effects from its advancement. More kids wearing eyeglasses will mean more adults who will go blind. It made me nervous just thinking about it.

When I returned to the office, the memory of that speech faded from my mind. That is until I sat in another symposium and the keynote speaker recalled the exact same lecture. But his experience when he returned to his office was very different. Several weeks afterward, he had developed "floaters," a visual phenomenon among many of our patients, especially those with myopia. And this doctor was indeed very nearsighted.

And then, a few weeks after the floaters appeared, his retina detached. As eye doctors we often feel immune to the disease that afflicts our patients. But we're not! My colleague, like so many other doctors, experienced the same sight threatening side effect of myopia. Luckily, these symptoms were recognized by the doctor and he got the treatment he needed in time. If he didn't know what to look for, he may have waited too long to avoid permanent vision loss.

There are three lessons here:

1) The best way to reduce the risk of blindness from myopia is to avoid it from developing in the first place. 2) Seek the care of your eye doctor immediately upon experiencing ANY changes to your vision. 3) Yearly eye exams are recommended to not only assure good vision, but healthy eyes!

Myopia is a disease that does not play favorites.

This is particularly noteworthy since projections have estimated over 1 billion people will suffer from the higher degree of myopia associated with these conditions.[3] Today, about one-fifth of young adults in East Asia have high myopia, and half of them are expected to develop irreversible vision loss, especially when they become older. If these trends continue, conservative estimates predict a sevenfold increase in irreversible vision loss by 2050. High myopes are not the only ones at risk. With only half the prescription the risk of retinal detachment is still significantly higher compared to those without myopia.[16]

To put this into perspective, the risk of glaucoma and cataracts due to myopia are the same as the risk of cardiovascular events due to untreated hypertension, as well as the risk of stroke from smoking 20 cigarettes per day![8] Even more alarming, the risk of retinal detachment and macular degeneration due to myopia are far in excess of any identified risk factor for cardiovascular disease![8]

The Myopia Epidemic is the Tip of the Iceberg!

In the 1970s when the prevalence of myopia was much lower, today's commonplace conveniences didn't exist. In the United States and other industrialized countries, children are brought up today with air conditioning, television, Internet, video games, and social media, all of which keeps them…indoors. I find tremendous irony in the correlation between the conveniences of modern life and the increased prevalence of childhood myopia. Irony? Why? Most parents work hard to provide the very conveniences that may be negatively affecting their children's eyesight, that's why!

More ominous than poor eyesight is the amount of pressure we inadvertently place on our children to perform academically. Since many children have more advantages growing up than their parents, it only makes sense that these same parents expect their children to exceed their own scholastic achievements.

I placed extraordinary expectations on my children, disproportionate to the ones placed on me as a child. When I was younger, I was expected to do well in school, but my life was balanced by playing with friends when I finished my homework. Today, scholastic competition among many teens has spiraled out of control.

The modern rise in myopia seems to mirror a trend for children to spend more time engaged in studying or, more recently, tethered to their computers and smartphones.

In addition, constant reliance on computers, tablets, and smartphones for information AND socialization keeps children indoors. Based on some studies on myopia, spending time indoors—especially in early childhood—induces the onset of myopia.[9] But exactly what is it about the outdoors that helps? Is it the bright sunlight? Is it that when we are outside our eyes focus on objects far away? Or is it something else entirely? We will look at the answers to some of these questions in upcoming chapters.

> There is no single cause for myopia, yet there are several ways to address it.

In summary, it is clear that myopia is on the rise and is associated with several sight-threatening conditions. And it's reaching epidemic proportions, especially among school-aged children. So why are most parents unaware of this threat to the safety and health of their kids? The purpose of this book is to educate parents, students, and teachers on the myopia epidemic and offer recommendations on how best to protect your child's vision. In the following pages, Dr. Noah Tannen delves deeper into the topic of myopia, what it is, why it occurs, and some of the traditional options used to correct it. He follows up in Part 3 with evidence-based research on ways doctors hope to slow myopia progression among students.

In Part 4, Kimberly Lee shares her experience both as a teacher and a mother challenged by her children's obsession with technology. In the final part, we wrap things up with pragmatic recommendations to parents. As you read, you may encounter terms that are technical or unfamiliar to you. Definitions and explanations of these terms can be found in Appendix A.

There is one thing I've learned examining children's vision for over three decades: there is no single cause for myopia, yet there are several ways to address it. The solution that's best for you and your child is derived from careful facts laid out within this book. I welcome you to benefit from our experience as caring professionals who happen to be parents, too!

A great sense of fulfillment comes from watching my young patients develop into productive adults. There is no greater feeling! Throughout the book, you'll find stories of some of these patients. These real life stories provide examples for the lessons presented in these pages. Each of these is shared with the permission of each family…including my own sons!

The Beginning

Noah Tannen

I realized medicine's approach to myopia may be "nearsighted," too.

Among my optometry school classmates, I was one of the lucky few. I didn't need glasses. Many students were children who spent their youth in and out of eye doctors' offices, but I was an anomaly.

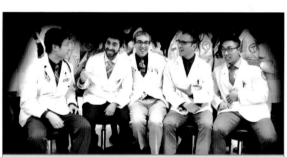

Dr. Noah (second from left) posing with classmates in optometry school

I was even called a "unicorn," a mythical student who doesn't need glasses or contact lenses. Believe it or not we actually do exist!

I was different from my colleagues since I was drawn to the field because I wanted to follow in my father's footsteps. When I was young I spent time in his office fascinated by all the equipment and gadgets in each exam room. I met his patients, listened to stories about how he had helped them and improved their quality of life. To me, it was an easy decision to join his proud profession. But why had most of my friends in school developed the need for glasses while I was spared?

I had always assumed that nearsightedness was inherited from your parents (my classmates must have been unlucky in the genetic vision lottery). My father has had perfect vision all of his life and I've heard enough "Mini-Me*" jokes to know that we share the same genes.

Multiple factors control whether someone develops nearsightedness.

My mother, on the other hand, has always been nearsighted. Like many people, my mother hates being dependent on her glasses, so she decided to try contact lenses. It didn't take long for my father to realize that family members can be the most difficult patients...but that's another story! While her attempt to wear contact lenses did not go as planned, it made it very clear to me that the traditional methods of correcting myopia were not enough for many patients.

Why were we treating the consequences of nearsightedness and not targeting the cause?

Luckily, my sister and I have been spared and neither of us needs glasses to see clearly. But if nearsightedness is genetic, shouldn't at least one of us require glasses? The more I learned about myopia, the more I realized this commonly-held belief was wrong. Like many things in life, multiple factors control whether someone develops nearsightedness.

As I came to this realization, I also began to see that medicine's approach to this common condition may be "nearsighted," too. There is more to a vision exam than simply asking, "Do you see better with lens one or lens two?" Why are we content with simply increasing the power of our young patients' glasses year after year, instead of actively trying to preserve their vision?

Why were we treating the consequences of nearsightedness and not targeting the cause?

*Mini-Me is a character in the Austin Powers movies, a clone of the main character who was identical in every way, but he was "one-eighth his size."

Correcting Myopia (Nearsightedness)

The first recorded distinction between nearsightedness and far-sightedness is often attributed to Aristotle in the 4th century BC. The

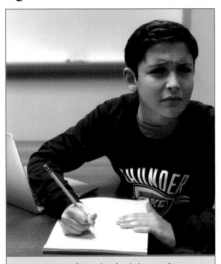

Nearsighted children have the tendency to squint, making their vision clearer without glasses, by creating a pinhole-like effect.

medical term for nearsighted-ness, *myopia*, comes from the Greek word *myopos*, or *myein,* meaning "too close," and *opos* meaning "eye."

Many of my young near-sighted patients develop a bad habit of squinting to see the school board or view an object at a distance. It's a natural ten-dency, but why does squinting work? Looking through a small hole in your fingers will work in a pinch when glasses are nowhere to be found. Let me show you what I mean. Take off your glasses (yes, right now).

Chances are you can't see very well across the room. That's okay; just pick a blurry object off in the distance. Now make a small hole with your index finger and thumb and look through it. Voila! It should now be clear!

This artificial pinhole, whether created by squinting your lids or a hole made by your fingers, decreases blur by eliminating the non-focusing peripheral light rays and concentrating on the clearest ones that fall on the retina at the back of the eye. Glasses, on the other hand, work by bending light rays toward a central focal point that lands precisely on the retina, providing a sharp image to the eye.

Interestingly, despite Aristotle's initial discovery over 2,000 years ago, the first known pair of eyeglasses was not invented until the end of the 13th century. These early glasses were mounted magnifying glasses held over reading material used to counteract *presbyopia*, or "old man eyes." The first eyeglasses for the correction of nearsightedness weren't invented until 150 years later, and it was another 250 years until side-arms (or temples) were added to frames allowing people to wear glasses on their face for the first time ever. Does that mean the nearsighted individuals Aristotle observed in Ancient Greece were destined for trades requiring sharp near acuity, otherwise squinting their way through a blurry life? Not exactly.

Despite most human populations abandoning the hunter-gatherer way of life long ago, a few of these isolated societies persisted into the early 20th century. Fortunately for us, these tribes provide a snapshot in time of the human condition before the advent and rise of modern technology. For instance, among the hunter-gatherer tribes of Gabon, formerly French Equatorial Africa, less than 1% of several thousand members are nearsighted. Similarly, low rates are found among the Angmagssalik Eskimos in Greenland.[10]

> These trends imply there is more at play than genetic factors alone.

The eyes of Inuits living in Alaska and the Northwest Territories of Canada, however, tell a different story. The older adults, who had lived most of their lives in isolated aboriginal communities, displayed similar rates of nearsightedness as the Angmagssalik Eskimos. However, the younger subjects, under the influence of increasing westernized acculturation and integration into American schooling, showed rates as high as 50%.[11]

These trends imply there is more at play than genetic factors alone. Clearly, some environmental changes precipitated the sudden rise in nearsightedness seen in the younger tribesmen that did not affect their parents.

Does Reading Negatively Impact Children's Eyesight?

For more than a century it has been assumed that excessive near work induces nearsightedness by causing the eyeball to elongate. This stretching of the eye causes light rays to fall short of the retina at the back of the eye. This long-held belief about near work is not incorrect, but it can be misleading. While it is well documented that excessive near work is correlated with nearsightedness, this does not provide the full picture.[12] Perhaps more detrimental than the near work itself is that it is performed indoors, away from natural light.

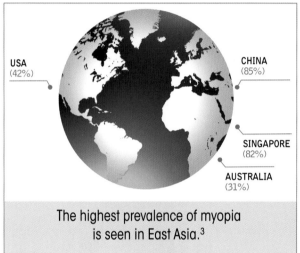

USA (42%)

CHINA (85%)

SINGAPORE (82%)

AUSTRALIA (31%)

The highest prevalence of myopia is seen in East Asia.[3]

Scientists now know that daily exposure to outdoor light protects against the development of nearsightedness.[13] While the young Inuit of Alaska and Canada did indeed read more than their parents, compulsory education also meant significantly less time outdoors. This is the real difference between the two generations.[13]

We can determine the role of each variable that may contribute to the development of myopia by comparing similar groups of people living different lifestyles. Researchers did exactly this in a cross-sectional study conducted in 2008.[14] Two groups of children were investigated in this study--both with the same genetic makeup. To be included in the study, both parents of the child had to be of Chinese descent. Between the two groups, there was no difference in the proportion of children with zero, one, or two nearsighted parents. The major difference between the groups, however, was that one group lived in Singapore, the other in Sydney, Australia. Despite having the same genetic makeup, ~30% of children living in Singapore versus 3% of those living in Sydney developed myopia.

What was the biggest factor accounting for this difference? The children in Sydney spent an average of 14 hours per week outdoors, while the children in Singapore spent only 3 hours. Interestingly, the children in Sydney actually spent more time reading, writing, or using computers compared to their Singaporean counterparts, yet still retained the protective benefits of spending more time outside.

What's Special About Being Outside?

The probability of a child becoming nearsighted by 14 years of age is around 60% if the child has two nearsighted parents and performs less than 5 hours per week of outdoor activity. This number drops to about 20% if that same child does at least 14 hours per week of outdoor activity. For every additional hour per week spent outdoors, there is a 2% reduction in the odds of developing nearsightedness. Exposure to the outdoors in youth virtually negates the genetic predisposition a child might have toward developing nearsightedness.[13]

> For every additional hour per week spent outdoors, there is a 2% reduction in the odds of developing nearsightedness.

Researchers have not yet arrived at a clear consensus on how being outside protects one's eyes from developing myopia, but many theories exist. The majority of daylight's protective benefits appear to lie in the intensity and wavelength composition of the outdoor light spectrum. Currently, the most widely-held belief is that natural daylight causes a release of dopamine in the eye, inhibiting eyeball growth and slowing down the progression of myopia.[15]

In addition to stimulating the release of dopamine in the eye, bright light causes pupil constriction. Pupil constriction acts as a natural pinhole to reduce image blur on the retina. Fewer blurry signals to the eye equal a slower rate of myopia progression.

Lastly, these benefits are compounded by farther viewing distances outdoors resulting in less demand to focus the eyes to see clearly. Excessive focusing of the eyes may cause nearsightedness to worsen.[16] Taken together, it's no surprise our daylight-dwelling ancestors didn't develop more nearsightedness.

Here is the problem today.

Not only are children learning to read at a younger age than their parents, they are facing ever-growing demands to perform well in school from a very young age. Add to this the meteoric rise of handheld electronics, and it's no wonder that children are spending significantly less time outdoors than their parents did.

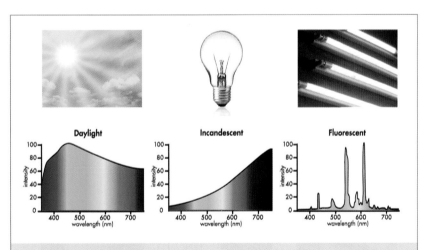

The properties of outdoor light have been found to be protective against the development of nearsightedness. Daylight emits high intensity light across all wavelengths of the electromagnetic spectrum. Artificial light is less intense and does not have as broad a spectrum of colors and wavelengths as natural light.

OUTDOOR PLAY

TYLER AND SAMANTHA'S STORY AS TOLD BY DR. D
Both have perfect 20/20 vision. Both parents are nearsighted.

Tyler and Samantha's mother was a teenager when I first examined her vision almost 30 years ago. She was fit with traditional hard contact lenses to correct her near-sightedness. At the time, myopia was considered hereditary and the thought of stopping its progression never came to mind. She wore her hard contacts until she had laser vision correction (LASIK) 20 years later.

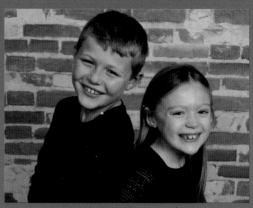

Tyler & Samantha

Tyler and Samantha's father has a high degree of myopia, so the odds that these children would one day wear eye-glasses was very high. However, Tyler, 10, and Samantha, 7, both have 20/20 vision. Is it luck? Will they inevitably need eyeglasses? I sense the answer lies in their household habits.

You see, their mom is a teacher, a very good one at that. At each of her eye examinations, we discuss how the lure of electronics affects the socialization of children. As a younger teacher she taught at different school districts; the more sought-after the district, the more technology was made available to students, and the more obsessed the children became with it.

To combat the trend she witnessed in her classroom, Ty and Sami were kept busy...very busy...balancing their lives outside of school. I spoke to their mom and asked if her children, who have perfect vision, play outside.

"I let them play outside right after school to burn off steam. Then they do home-work, then dinner and then the fun begins! In the fall, both kids practice soccer during the week and have games on the weekend. In the spring, they play baseball and softball, with pretty much the same routine. In the summer we LIVE outside! We LOVE summertime! The kids swim in their grandmother's pool, go to the beach, play in the backyard, and ride their bikes. Summer is family time!

"So during those three seasons, electronic use is definitely limited because we just don't have the time. They'd rather play outside with friends or participate in sports than be indoors. Winter, however, is another story. Both play basketball, but overall winter is our indoor time. We don't limit their electronic use probably as much as we should. We've looked up age-appropriate restrictions. They both got a tablet for Christmas, but during the week we've started a 1-hour limit on their electronics, in addition to whatever homework requires computers."

We know from the Sydney Myopia Study[14] that playing outdoors is protective against the progression of myopia, and may even negate the risk of nearsightedness from excessive close work. How much time outdoors is needed? Scientists are not sure, but some say as little as 45 minutes per day may help and that's just helping their eyesight!

What about the winter months when outdoor play is limited? It's no surprise that children's myopia may tend to progress more at that time of year than in the summer months.[53] Perhaps Ty and Sami were spared due to the limits their mother placed on screen time during the colder months. I encourage her to follow her maternal and professional instincts to limit their screen time and continually encourage the children to entertain themselves outdoors. I'm also quick to remind her that once bad eyesight starts, it's difficult to arrest it, since outdoor time does not seem to reverse myopia progression. I close with this silly proverb: "An hour outside per day...keeps the eye doctor away!"

Although, sunlight is important in prevention, its benefit once myopia develops is unclear. Recent evidence may indicate that there is some residual benefit to outdoor activities for children who are nearsighted.[17] However, the consensus is once myopia starts, it becomes more difficult to slow down. It's like a boulder rolling down a hill, picking up momentum. The younger the child develops myopia, the more rapidly their eyesight deteriorates, increasing the likelihood a side effect from myopia will occur in their lifetime.

It is time to abandon the traditional view of nearsighted correction in favor of nearsighted prevention.

For those children who do spend ample time outdoors, it is important to remember that sunlight can be both beneficial and harmful if proper precautions aren't taken. This means that children still need sunscreen and sunglasses to protect their skin and eyes from potentially harmful UV radiation while outdoors.

Which Is Better: Reading From a Tablet or Book?

I'm frequently asked if reading from paper books has less impact on vision when compared to performing work on computers, tablets, and smartphones. The honest answer is we really don't know. Doctors have theories, but science-based research has not caught up with the onslaught of electronics used to read, write, and communicate.

My personal belief is that electronics have an addictive nature not found among other tasks performed up close, like reading, sewing, or origami. We discuss this in more detail toward the end of the book, but it makes sense; the more we and our children are online, the less time they get outside and the more likely myopia will develop and progress. Bottom line, screens keep us stationary, they keep us from moving. We don't have to go the library or bookstore, we can download book after book without lifting our heads.

It should also be noted that people blink as much as 80% less while using electronic devices.[54] This phenomenon has been attributed to the brightness of the screen. In fact, people also blink significantly less when looking into a fire. Reduced blink rate means the tear film is not renewed and the eyes dry out more quickly. In severe cases, chronic dryness can even cause damage to the cornea. More and more, our young patients who spend excessive time on screens are complaining of chronic dry eye; a trend we did not observe prior to the widespread use of electronics.

What about the light that radiates from screens? Scientists are uncertain if the radiation emitted from screens harms our eyesight or increases the risk of certain eye diseases. But, the American Academy of Pediatrics recommends that children younger than 18 months get ZERO time with a screen, and those aged 2 to 5 years should be limited to 30 minutes a day. This is half of its prior recommendation.

I prefer that all elementary school children avoid electronics totally during the school week since they get enough screen time at or after school. They need to learn to relax or decompress in some other way than with electronics. We'll make this clearer in the following sections of our book.

So How SHOULD Nearsightedness Be Corrected?

There are many ways doctors are trying to stop children's eyesight from worsening once myopia develops. Currently, the most effective treatments include:

1. Orthokeratology, special overnight contact lenses worn while the child sleeps that are removed in the morning
2. Multifocal contact lenses worn during the day and removed at night
3. A nightly eye drop called atropine

The most challenging aspect is convincing clinicians and parents that it is time to abandon the traditional view of nearsighted correction, replace it with nearsighted prevention, and move in favor of a healthier option to stop this epidemic from spreading.

Putting on the Brakes

Noah Tannen

Inform, educate, and recommend.

After graduating from optometry school, I elected to complete a residency in pediatrics and vision rehabilitation. One of the requirements for completion was to give a presentation, which was open to all doctors and students at the institution. I chose childhood myopia as my subject. While this topic has received significant interest in recent years, it wasn't a mainstream topic back when I was a resident and I was feeling apprehensive about the subject I had chosen.

Would others find the topic as interesting as I did?

Would professionals outside of the pediatric department benefit from the information?

Do doctors already know about the epidemic of myopia among children, but choose to ignore it?

Much to my delight, the presentation was a hit! However, it soon became clear that not only were doctors failing to incorporate measures to prevent myopia at the university, many didn't even know how to do so. While many in attendance were aware that strategies existed, few were familiar with the research or specifics regarding how to implement these treatments.

Soon after my presentation, the president of the university approached me and asked how myopia control could be better implemented into the clinics. Myopia prevention or control was not practiced at our university and our unintended inaction was failing to help a staggering number of children. So, together, we created a plan to incorporate modern myopia treatments into the routine clinical care of our pediatric patients. The first myopia control clinic in the country was developed by Maria Liu, OD, PhD, at the University Eye Center, UC Berkeley; and today there are several optometry schools that offer this service to concerned parents. It was also a catalyst for me and I now conduct both continuing education lectures for eye doctors, as well as online courses for students, to spread awareness and education about myopia prevention and methods to slow down its progression.

There is still a lot of work to do. Even though more research is being conducted on treatments and methods to stop or slow down the progression of myopia, only one-third of community eye doctors actively incorporate myopia control into their routine clinical care today.[18] While encouraging research is great news, we are far from the finish line. In fact, none of the treatments currently available in the United States are FDA (Food and Drug Administration) approved to slow down nearsightedness, only to correct it. Despite the absence of FDA approval, there is a plethora of evidence-based research that supports several effective myopia control treatments.[19] Research has shown that there are several ways to possibly slow down the progression of myopia but it's up to the individual eye doctor and parent to decide how best to proceed. That's the purpose of this chapter: inform, educate, and recommend.

> While encouraging research is great news, we are far from the finish line.

What is 20/20 Vision Anyway?

Visual acuity is quantified by a chart such as the one to the right. Most people think of vision in terms of 20/20, 20/70, 20/200, etc. But what does that mean? In simplified terms, the numerator of this fraction refers to the testing dis-

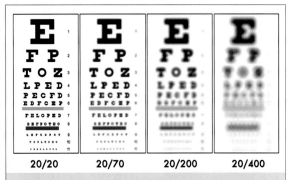

The appearance of a standard Snellen eye chart from 20 feet away with varying degrees of visual acuity. A student with 20/20 vision sees much clearer than a child with 20/400 vision.

tance, or 20 feet by convention. The denominator refers to the size of the letter that can be seen from this testing distance. If a person can see the 20/20 letter from 20 feet away, that person has 20/20 (or average) vision. A person who can only see the 20/70 letter from 20 feet away has 20/70 vision. The big "E" on this eye chart is 20/200. This means that a normally sighted person can stand 200 feet away and see this letter, but someone with 20/200 vision has to stand 20 feet away from it. Many of the children I examine with nearsightedness cannot see the big "E" at the top of the eye chart without the use of eyeglasses. To me, that's not only bothersome, it's alarming.

During vision exams, refractive conditions including myopia are quantified with a term called "diopters" denoted by a "D." A diopter is a unit of measurement that denotes the power of an optical device, such as a spectacle lens or the human eye. The higher the degree of myopia, the worse a person sees at a distance and the higher the diopter value in the prescription. A child with a prescription of -2.00D sees blurrier at a distance than a child with a prescription of -1.00D. For those children who develop nearsightedness, the average rate of progression during adolescence is about -0.50 diopter per year.[20] So, if a child begins to develop nearsightedness around age six, by the time he or she is eighteen, the child can easily reach at least -6.00 diopters of nearsightedness…unless there is intervention. Greater than -5.00D is

Myopia is MUCH more than an inconvenience.

considered high nearsightedness and considerably increases the risk of blindness from a side effect of myopia, including retinal detachment, macular degeneration, and glaucoma, as mentioned in the earlier chapter. Myopia is MUCH more than an inconvenience. The World Health Organization predicts more than 1 billion people will suffer from this higher degree of myopia by 2050, placing them in jeopardy of losing their vision as they age.[21]

Myopia is not to be confused with astigmatism, which is a big, scary, word. However, astigmatism simply means the eye's surface isn't completely spherical. Almost all of us have astigmatism to some degree. While both myopia and astigmatism may cause blur, the degree of astigmatism does not tend to increase yearly.

Unfortunately, at this time there is no treatment or strategy available to guarantee complete arrest of the progression of nearsightedness, but with current methods we can significantly slow it down and ideally stabilize the child into a low-risk category.

What is Myopia Control?

While there is no known cure for myopia, there are now a number of treatments available to "control" myopia. In other words, to slow down the progression of nearsightedness so your child does not need a stronger pair of glasses year after year. This is achieved through the clinical application of eyeglasses, contact lenses, and/or eye drops.

Why Don't Eyeglasses or Traditional Contact Lenses Stop Myopia?

Glasses and traditional contact lenses work by focusing light rays on the retina at the back of the eye. This provides clear central vision.

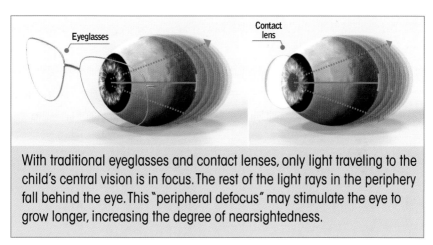

With traditional eyeglasses and contact lenses, only light traveling to the child's central vision is in focus. The rest of the light rays in the periphery fall behind the eye. This "peripheral defocus" may stimulate the eye to grow longer, increasing the degree of nearsightedness.

The remainder of the light rays, however, land behind the retina in the periphery, referred to as "peripheral defocus." We don't notice these peripheral rays of light because the blur caused by them is in our peripheral vision. Researchers now know that peripheral defocus appears to stimulate the eye to grow longer, making the eye even more nearsighted.[5]

When my father trained as an optometrist, many believed children should remove their eyeglasses while reading to stop myopia from getting worse. The prevailing theory was that excessive focusing of the eyes caused the prescription to worsen and removing the glasses caused children to focus their eyes less while reading. Unfortunately, while the logic seemed sound, this method failed to work. In fact, researchers found that removing eyeglasses not only fails to work, but this continuous under correction may actually accelerate the myopic prescription.[22] Bifocal eyeglasses, where the bottom of the lens contains a prescription specifically for reading, also failed to stabilize the prescription.[23*]   The reason is because these interventions do not eliminate peripheral defocus over a large enough area of the retina.

So, theoretically, if peripheral defocus or blur can be eliminated across a larger portion of the retina, it can stop myopia from worsening. The good news is we can do it! Currently, two types of specialty contact lenses exist to curtail nearsightedness by reducing peripheral defocus over a larger area of the retina: multifocal daytime contact lenses and overnight-wear, corneal reshaping contact lenses (orthokeratology).[24,25]

Contact Lenses Designed to Slow Down Myopia

Multifocal or bifocal contact lenses provide both distance and reading correction in a single lens. These soft contact lenses were initially designed for patients over the age of 40 who have trouble reading up close. For myopia control patients, a lens with center distance correction and a near correction in the periphery enables the central light rays to fall correctly on the retina and also focuses the peripheral light rays on the retina.

Reducing blur across the entire visual field has been shown to be effective at slowing down the progression of nearsightedness. According to current research, the prescription can be slowed by about 30% to 50% with these lenses.[24]

> So, theoretically, if peripheral defocus or blur can be eliminated across a larger portion of the retina, it can stop myopia from worsening. The good news is we can do it!

It should be noted, however, that some small subsets of children did appear to benefit. This included children with poor eye focusing skills (accommodative insufficiency) and the tendency for their eyes to turn inward during near work (esophoria). Unfortunately, in a follow-up study, researchers were unable to reproduce the benefits noted among those with focusing and eye coordination issues.[34] While bifocal glasses might be helpful for some children, they do not appear to slow down myopia for the vast majority of nearsighted patients.

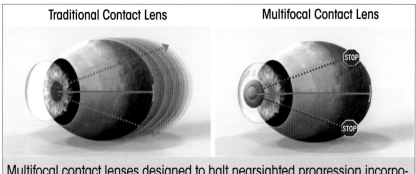

Traditional Contact Lens **Multifocal Contact Lens**

Multifocal contact lenses designed to halt nearsighted progression incorporate a myopia prevention zone (red) to minimize peripheral defocus, while the central vision (green) remains fully corrected (myopia correction).

While soft multifocal contact lenses are generally comfortable and well tolerated, even by younger patients, it is important that the child wears the lenses during all waking hours in order to prevent myopia from progressing. Children may complain of dry eyes because the lenses are worn all day long. They may also notice glare and some blurry vision because of the presence of multiple prescriptions within the multifocal contact lens. It can be a challenge for the patient and the doctor, balancing the visual and physical comfort of the patient on a day-to-day basis, with the goal of controlling the progression of myopia over the long term. That's why my first choice of treatment is a contact lens that is worn while the child sleeps, called *orthokeratology*.

Lenses Designed to Correct Vision While You Sleep?

Orthokeratology contact lenses can be referred to by many names, making it confusing for parents. They may be referred to as "OK lens," "corneal molding," "corneal reshaping," "ortho-k," "gentle vision shaping," as well as by trademarked names by individual manufacturers. Regardless of the name, these contact lenses work by

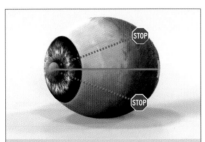

Orthokeratology lenses reshape the front of the eye (cornea) while the child sleeps at night. Upon removal in the morning, both the myopia correction (green) and prevention (red) zones imprinted on the eye last all day. This allows the child to see clearly without the use of daytime contacts or eyeglasses.

reshaping the curve on the front of the eye (the cornea) while the patient sleeps to provide clear vision the next day without the need for contact lenses or eyeglasses. The contact lens itself does not have a corrective prescription like a standard or multifocal contact lens, although it does allow clear vision while it is being worn. The vision is corrected by actually reshaping the cornea to allow light rays to focus precisely on the back of the eye, or central retina.

The cornea can maintain its new

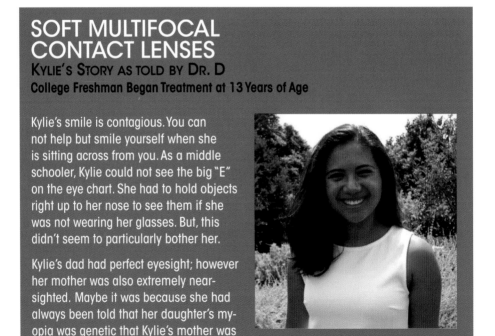

SOFT MULTIFOCAL CONTACT LENSES
KYLIE'S STORY AS TOLD BY DR. D
College Freshman Began Treatment at 13 Years of Age

Kylie's smile is contagious. You can not help but smile yourself when she is sitting across from you. As a middle schooler, Kylie could not see the big "E" on the eye chart. She had to hold objects right up to her nose to see them if she was not wearing her glasses. But, this didn't seem to particularly bother her.

Kylie's dad had perfect eyesight; however her mother was also extremely near-sighted. Maybe it was because she had always been told that her daughter's myopia was genetic that Kylie's mother was relentless in finding a treatment that

Kylie

would potentially stop her daughter's eyesight from getting worse. Referred by a friend, they traveled over an hour to visit our office to see if we could help.

Our first choice was overnight orthokeratology lenses, but Kylie's prescription was too strong, eliminating this option. The next possibility was soft multifocal or bifocal contact lenses. These lenses not only provide clear vision during the time they are worn, the periphery of the lens also helps stop or slow down myopia from getting worse.

Kylie's parents pondered carefully, taking several weeks to make a decision. They had been told by previous eye care doctors that there was nothing that could be done to stop their daughter's eyesight from getting worse. They needed science, articles, and tests to be sure. Finally, after reassurance from us, they started the treatment for their daughter.

I verified that while genetics does indeed play a role in children developing myopia or nearsightedness, environment also plays a role. This was not difficult for Kylie's parents to understand; their daughter was a stellar student who loved to read…and read…and read…!

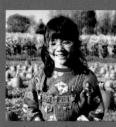

Kylie is now a college freshman, majoring in journalism. Her vision has not gotten worse since we fit her with soft multifocal contact lenses. Kylie's self-esteem and (dare I say) quality of life have also improved by getting rid of her thick eyeglasses and wearing contact lenses instead. We've reduced her risk of developing sight-threatening conditions associated with high degrees of myopia. Kylie and her parents (and her optometrist) have the confidence that everything possible was done to preserve her eyesight as she enters this next

Kylie with glasses level of scholastic demand.

curve for 12 to 24 hours after being reshaped by these orthokeratology contact lenses and then it will slowly return to its original curvature. In fact, within one week of discontinuing lens wear, most of the positive effect of the lens will have completely worn off. Therefore, these lenses must be worn nightly, often for many years, until the prescription is stable.

Even though these contact lenses are rigid, they are generally better tolerated than soft lenses since they are only worn during sleep, as opposed to all waking hours. Orthokeratology also appears to have a slightly greater impact on the slowing of myopia than multifocal soft contact lenses, giving it additional benefits.[19]

But is it safe to sleep in contact lenses?

You may have heard that contact lenses should not be worn while sleeping, even though the FDA has approved several types of contact lenses for overnight wear, including those for orthokeratology. Fortunately, the material used for orthokeratology contact lenses is highly permeable to the oxygen that is greatly needed by the cornea. Also, as long as proper hygiene and instructions are followed, the disinfection process for these contact lenses is very effective at eliminating harmful bacteria. A recent large-scale study reported the incidence of serious infection to be less than 8 infections per 10,000 years of wear among orthokeratology lens wearers.[26] Long-term success of treatment requires a combination of proper lens fitting, rigorous compliance to the lens care regimen, good adherence to routine follow-ups, and timely treatment of complications.

While orthokeratology contact lenses are generally well tolerated, patients may experience other side effects about which they should be thoroughly educated before proceeding. Some wearers might complain of glare or halos around lights at night. Generally, this glare does not affect vision, but may be bothersome, especially while driving at night. While this is not an issue in younger patients, many children will continue to wear these lenses throughout college and graduate school. In fact, continuation of wear is encouraged as the prescription is still liable to change as long as the individual spends prolonged periods of time reading and studying. When glare cannot be eliminated completely, we transition to a different form of correction, like traditional contact lenses, and monitor the wearer closely.

Since these contact lenses work by flattening the central cornea, there is also the potential to cause irritation in that area. Signs of irritation include pain, redness, tearing, discharge, visual distortion, and even ocular abrasion. Fortunately, patients using this modality

ORTHOKERATOLOGY CONTACT LENSES
EMILY'S STORY AS TOLD BY HER MOTHER
High School Freshman Began Treatment at 11 Years of Age

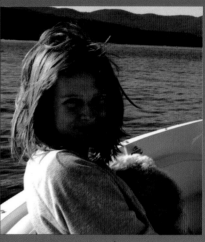

Emily

Within a space of 6 months, my 11-year-old daughter, Emily, went from being far-sighted to suddenly finding herself diagnosed with progressive myopia. She was very upset at the prospect of having to wear glasses and we were desperate to prevent her vision from deteriorating further. Emily's developmental optometrist told us about a few options, with ortho-keratology being the most promising. While she had her doubts that my daughter would adjust to the lenses, we were determined to explore this option, so we booked an appointment with Dr. Lee at Dr. D's office.

Dr. Lee was friendly and professional; within minutes he was laughing and joking with Emily. The program was explained to us with the level of technical detail I needed in order to understand how it all worked. Emily was evaluated and found to be a good candidate for orthokeratology lenses. We made the commitment and embarked on a new adventure.

One of the technicians in the practice did a splendid job of getting Emily familiar with the lenses, as well as teaching her how to apply and remove them efficiently and safely. She gave us tips and loads of encouragement. During the training session, Emily managed quickly to apply the lenses and all seemed to be going well. That lasted until we arrived home to do it on our own. It was a steep learning curve and at one point I even thought of throwing in the towel. Emily would have none of it. She was determined to persevere!

All through the learning process, the staff and doctors were available to help and guide us. We went back for a few extra teaching sessions. Emily was off and running! She immediately loved her perfect vision during the day and I was especially thrilled to learn later that her myopia had not progressed. She is now 3 years into the program and it's nothing but smooth sailing. She independently applies and removes her lenses, cleans them and takes care of them without assistance, and has not yet lost a lens. We are all very happy.

are monitored very closely and modifications can be made to the contact lenses if these problems arise. Doctors fitting these contact lenses should maintain constant communication with their patients in order to address these problems before they become serious. It is important to find a clinician with experience fitting multiple types of orthokeratology contact lenses to ensure he or she can choose the best lens for your individual child's eyes.

> It is important to find a clinician with experience fitting multiple types of orthokeratology contact lenses to ensure he or she can choose the best lens for your individual child's eyes.

Both of Dr. Despotidis' sons were fit with orthokeratology lenses, shortly after being diagnosed with myopia almost 20 years ago. His son Nicholas continues to wear the lenses as he approaches 30 years of age. After college, children fit with this technology are given the option to transition to eyeglasses or contact lenses, however the majority choose to continue into adulthood. Dr. D's younger son discontinued orthokeratology shortly after college. The goal of stabilizing his eyesight was achieved and his work and graduate demands interfered with the consistent wearing required with orthokeratology. His younger son now wears eyeglasses and soft contact lenses socially and luckily his vision has not changed since he discontinued four years ago. His ultimate goal is to permanently correct his eyesight with LASIK eye surgery after he's completed medical school. So, how long are orthokeratology lenses worn? The answer is until you and your doctor decide when the benefit of technology is outweighed by the demands of your lifestyle. In our office we ask students to continue wearing their orthokeratology lenses until their academic demands slow down significantly, normally after college.

OVERNIGHT ORTHOKERATOLOGY LENSES
ERIC'S STORY AS TOLD BY DR. D
Fifth Grader Began Treatment at 7 Years of Age

Eric is an extremely bright young man. He was referred to us by his family optometrist, since his myopia was progressing at a rapid pace. His prescription had already progressed to the point he could not see the big "E" on the eye chart without eyeglasses, and his myopia showed no sign of slowing down. He was only in second grade.

I should have realized Eric was not your ordinary seven-year-old when he correctly named most parts of the eye on the model eyeball I keep in my exam room! He was familiar with the eyeball, comfortable in an eye care office, and to Eric, wearing eyeglasses was not an inconvenience.

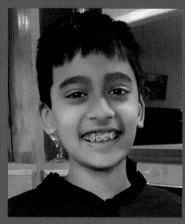

Eric

However, his mother was determined her son's eyesight would not be in jeopardy any longer. So, we decided on a treatment including overnight orthokeratology lenses. When we attempted to apply these special contacts, Eric was overwhelmed. He could not manage his fear. He simply refused.

Eric is a smart young man. However, wearing contact lenses, even to be slept in, was too much work. AND he had to put the lenses in his eyes EVERY night?? No way!!

So, instead we prescribed diluted atropine eye drops. Eric's mother instilled one drop in each of his eyes every night. She filled the prescription at a special compound pharmacy that diluted the drop to a safe, yet effective, level. We adjusted the dosage of the atropine drop until Eric's vision stabilized. Weeks turned into months. Eric even learned to put the drops in all by himself. Everyone was happy!

A year later, Eric surprised me by saying, "Dr. D, I'd like to try the overnight lenses again. I think I can do it this time."

Apprehensive but excited, my staff prepared a diagnostic pair of lenses for Eric's

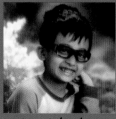

eyes. It was as if a magical spell came over Eric and the office. He not only allowed our technician to apply the special lenses, he actually smiled with joy!

That was 18 months ago. Eric successfully wears his overnight contact lenses to maintain 20/20 vision during the day without eyeglasses or daytime contact lenses. His mother and I decided to maintain the atropine eye drops at night, as an added protection, until Eric reaches adolescence.

Eric with glasses

Nightly Eye Drops

While there are specialty contact lenses that are effective at slowing the myopia progression, they are not the best option for everyone. Some children cannot tolerate contact lenses, others may fail to properly care for them, and some may simply be too young.

There is an alternate treatment in the form of a nightly eye drop called atropine. Atropine is traditionally used to dilate the eyes and treat certain eye conditions. More recently, researchers have shown atropine to be effective at controlling the progression of nearsightedness, even when used in small doses.[27]

While there are theories as to how atropine works to slow myopia progress, the true mechanism remains unclear and atropine, like other methods we've discussed, is considered an off-label treatment. That means that this FDA-approved drug is used for a non-approved treatment.

Several studies point to atropine as the most effective treatment currently available.[19] Unfortunately, this medication comes with downsides. Even in its diluted form, atropine may produce side effects such as light sensitivity, glare, near vision blur, and allergic reaction.

The use of atropine to control the progression of myopia remains promising as research and studies continue. As there are currently challenges for its mainstream use, we support the use of atropine only for short-term use until the child is ready to transition to contact lenses, or as combination therapy in cases where contact lenses fail to work adequately.

What is the Best Age to Start Myopia Control?

It's simple: intervention should be initiated as soon as there is any indication of nearsightedness. Many studies confirm that age of onset is the strongest predictor of the development of high nearsightedness later

NIGHTLY ATROPINE DROPS
ZACHARY AND SARAH'S STORY AS TOLD BY DR. D
Eighth and Fifth Grader Respectively
Both Began Treatment at 9 Years of Age

Zachary was 6 years old when he first came to us as a patient. He sat motionless in my exam chair. I asked if he had trouble seeing the white board at school and his response was a quick, "NO!" This is common among younger students. In elementary school, the classroom is normally small in size and the amount of board work is often kept to a minimum. So, Zachary was "asymptomatic" in doctor-speak.

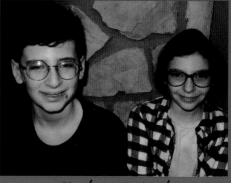

Zachary & Sarah

Yet, his exam revealed that Zachary was indeed slightly nearsighted. I noted this in my record, and proceeded to educate his parents on the need for him to limit electronic devices and encourage Zachary to play outside. His parents nodded in strong agreement. However, six months later, Zachary's eyeglass prescription more than doubled. He was destined to develop severe myopia as an adult, exposing to him to sight-threatening conditions, like retinal detachment.

At his appointment, I gently asked little Zachary, "Would you like to wear contact lenses?" He turned pale. Just the thought of touching his eye made him shiver with fear. He wanted to make his parents happy by trying them on, but thinking about it scared him.

"Would you let mom or dad place a drop in your eye to help stop your eyesight from getting worse?" He turned to his parents with despair, "If I have to!"

Zachary's parents, like many parents (maybe even you), had a lot of questions about atropine drops and its use. Were they safe? Do other eye doctors prescribe them? How do they work? Are there side effects? We created a handout for parents like Zachary's who are interested in atropine eye drops for myopia control. We've included a copy in Appendix C.

Fast forward one year and Zachary's eyesight is stable. But it has not been easy. We evaluate his vision every few months and increase the dosage ever so slightly, until we sense his eyesight has stopped changing. At each visit, we check for potential side effects, which may include light sensitivity and blurred vision while reading. We are happy to report that Zachary and most of our patients have experienced none of these!

The story does not end here. Zachary's younger sister, Sarah, developed nearsightedness when she reached the 3rd grade. Genetics are a very powerful contributor to myopia, in addition to environment. Like her brother, Sarah was NOT interested in orthokeratology contact lenses. We again recommended atropine eye drops.

Now, both Zachary and Sarah look forward to their visits and neither they nor their parents experience anxiety concerning their vision possibly worsening. Instead, the focus is on compliance and of course....reminding everyone of the importance of playing outside and limiting the use of electronics.

in life.[28] The younger a child is when myopia develops, the more likely they are to aggressively progress as they mature. In my opinion, a child is never too young to start treatment.

> It's simple; intervention should be initiated as soon as there is any indication of nearsightedness.

Exercises and Natural Remedies

While there are many different forms of eye exercises available to patients, currently no research supports their effectiveness at slowing the myopic progression.*

Some clinicians train patients to relax the focus of their eyes, which may also reduce nearsightedness, referring to this as vision therapy. Due to the lack of solid research for these methods, they should not be the first line of treatment. However, vision therapy may be

*NOTE: The "Bates Method" and the "See Clearly Method" are two exercise remedies that are advertised to improve eyesight and eliminate the need for glasses. It should be noted that these techniques have been debunked and do not improve vision or stop the prescription from worsening. Nor does the practice of "eye rubbing" or "acupressure eye exercises." If not done correctly, these procedures may even be dangerous or damage the eyes further. We do not endorse or recommend any of these remedies to improve eyesight and any doctor who does should be met with skepticism.

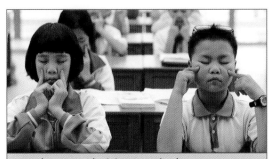

Chinese children rub their eyes to improve vision, but no benefit has been found to prevent myopia.

beneficial for another purpose. Certain eye coordination and focusing issues (specifically *convergence excess* and *accommodative insufficiency*) may contribute to the development of nearsightedness. Working with children to fix the underlying eye coordination problem may indeed slow the progression of nearsightedness, especially when used in conjunction with other methods we've already discussed. Specialty contact lenses and atropine remain the most effective modality for reducing the progression of nearsightedness over time.

> Specialty contact lenses and atropine remain the most effective modality for reducing the progression of nearsightedness over time.

The Future Looks Bright

As the epidemic continues to worsen, significant attention and research has been done in the area of controlling nearsightedness. Some countries like China, Taiwan, and Singapore have already implemented public policy measures in an effort to curb the growing rates of nearsightedness. For instance, Singapore has implemented "nature kindergartens" where children have most of their classes outdoors in an effort to maximize sun exposure.[29] China has even experimented with schools made entirely of glass to allow as much daylight in as possible during the school day.[29] The Chinese

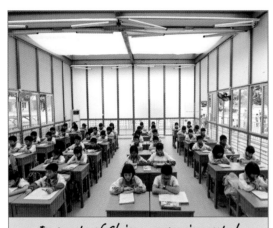

In parts of China, experimental "outdoor classrooms" have been constructed to maximize daily light exposure, in hopes of deterring myopia development in students.

government has made it illegal for a child under two years old to use an electronic device.[30] In the United States, the American Academy of Pediatrics recommends parents avoid exposing their children to electronics, like tablets and smartphones, before the age of two.[31]

Even so, these measures are likely not enough to stop this epidemic. Fortunately, new technologies are on the horizon that have the potential to significantly reduce nearsightedness worldwide. One such technology that may be available in the coming years utilizes the principles of multifocal soft contact lenses, but in the form of overnight wear orthokeratology lenses. It is expected that combining the effective properties of both modalities will work synergistically to reduce nearsightedness progression.

More exciting is the development of drug-dispensing contact lenses. These novel contact lenses will combine the designs already used for controlling nearsightedness, but will add a drug delivery system that dispenses continuous atropine or a drug with similar effects.[32] In fact, both of these technologies already exist but are still under investigation. It will likely take several more

As the epidemic continues to worsen, significant attention and research has been done in the area of controlling nearsightedness.

years until these treatments are commercially available.

Until then, my strong recommendation is to seek an eye care professional who views myopia with the same seriousness as you do. Remember, there are many researched methods to help your child, if the need arises. Parents must seek eye professionals familiar with the available treatments while being empathetic to your concerns.

One day, we might even have a cure for nearsightedness in the form of gene therapy. Researchers are working hard to identify the genes that control nearsightedness and modify those genes directly to eliminate nearsightedness.[33] Unfortunately, this research is still in its infancy and studies have not yet progressed past animal models. Nonetheless, this remains an exciting prospect with a great deal of potential in the future.

> Fortunately, new technologies are on the horizon that have the potential to significantly reduce nearsightedness worldwide.

Most importantly, allow your kids to play outdoors, something easier said than done, as my co-author Kim Lee discusses in our next section.

Through a Mother's Eyes

Kimberly Lee

Where Are All the Children?

Up until now, discussion has revolved around myopia development, available treatments to correct it, and perhaps even prevent its
progression among children. But as a mother of three and a school
teacher, my focus runs deeper than preserving eyesight. My sole purpose is to help raise healthy, well-adjusted children…a mission that's
become increasingly more difficult in the "digital world."

Here is my story…

I met my husband, Ivan, in college and we wed shortly after he became an optometrist. As an aspiring teacher, I remember envisioning
raising our children with a strong set of family values, like honesty
and respect. I believed the steps necessary to realizing those goals
were chatting during meals, encouraging my children to develop
friendships with "good" kids around the neighborhood, and overall…just laughing together! At the time, I could have never imagined the impact technology would have on those ideals. The
challenge became vividly clear after our first child began elementary school.

When our son developed myopia, it was not much of a concern;
my husband practices with Dr. Despotidis, and he immediately fit
my son, Tristan, with special night-time orthokeratology contacts. At
the time, I did not know much about them; that was my husband's

expertise and I trusted he was doing everything possible to preserve our son's eyesight. Honestly, I don't even recall making an association between Tristan's increasing time spent indoors with his deteriorating eyesight. Like most parents, my youth was spent outdoors. The action was always outside! But now, electronics brought the outdoors inside.

As a young teacher, my focus was in establishing a classroom environment that nurtured relationships: where academics came second to character development. I spent Septembers establishing routines and creating bonds between students through team building activities. The more time and work spent on character development, the less conflict I encountered throughout the year. My students experienced the joy of learning, without academic pressure. They could take risks, fail, and knew their peers and teacher would support them. Limited conflicts between classmates translated into a faster academic pace.

Not being a parent at the start of my career, I regret now the amount of homework I gave. Although my assignments were developmentally appropriate, I did not realize then how difficult it is for families to accomplish homework in the few short hours between after school and bedtime. Families rarely sit down to dinner together. For some families, homework can put a real strain on the parent/child relationship.

My educational philosophy drove us to find a school environment that made character development a priority. We did not want to move to a school district where increasing academic pressure and competition would keep our children inside studying for hours each day. We wanted a balanced education; access to honors and AP classes, yet equal access to clubs, sports and service organizations. Although we expect our children to work hard on their studies, we also wanted them to have time to exercise, relax, and enjoy meals with us. To us, success in life does not start with the highest GPA. Having well balanced children who are social, engaged and empathetic to others was a goal more important than class valedictorian.

So, when we were young newlyweds, we began searching for our first home. I was teaching 1st grade in a prominent school district; my husband, Ivan, was starting his career as an optometrist. We were looking for two things in our new home: close proximity to work and a highly-ranked school district. The community where we found our home was known for amazing standardized test scores and high academic rankings. We were certain we had found our perfect fit.

We loved our little townhome in our quiet little neighborhood. But after our children were born we noticed something…unusual. Every morning and afternoon, we saw groups of school-aged youngsters lugging heavy backpacks to and from the bus stop. But, in the afternoon, the playground was deserted. On long walks around our neighborhood, I rarely saw other mothers out and about with their kids.

Where were all the children?

The children in my neighborhood were growing up with easy access to electronics, computers, the Internet, and cell phones. Were they all inside…staring at screens? According to Jean M. Twenge in her book *iGen: Why Today's Super-Connected Kids Are Growing Up Less Rebellious, More Tolerant, Less Happy — and Completely Unprepared for Adulthood — and What That Means for the Rest of Us*, the iGen (children born in 1995 or later) had arrived.[35]

We wanted to find a community that would encompass our values.

We wanted to live in an excellent school district, but was there so much academic pressure for high test scores that children were tethered to their homework? We began to reconsider where we had chosen to raise our family.

And so, the search for a home began again. This time we wanted to find a community that would encompass our values. We wanted a neighborhood that nurtured social interaction, outdoor play, accessibility to stores and schools, and still had a strong school system. We found just that in an old-fashioned town covering a single square mile. Instead of a desert of isolation, we found an oasis of life. The main street was alive with people of all ages; couples were strolling, children were buzzing by on bikes, teens were devouring slices on the sidewalk in front of the pizza parlour. Some residents were shopping, others sunning themselves on benches, still others petting their dogs while chatting with shopkeepers. Everything about this town encouraged people to walk, socialize, and build relationships. The local grammar school, library, town hall, grocery store, bank, ice cream parlor, coffee shop, and sushi restaurant were all within walking distance of the homes lining the main street. There were parks, an organic farm, woods, hiking and biking trails, an equestrian center, and a fishing pond all reachable by bike. We had found a community that would keep our kids engaged and encourage a love of the outdoors....or so we hoped.

As parents we saw value in our children growing up with a lot of outdoor play and limited electronic use. We had noticed that when our young children had access to screen time, they became irritable, bleary eyed, non-communicative, and detached from reality. Both of our kids would ignore us when they were watching TV or playing on a tablet. They had trouble stopping when asked to turn off their games. We saw the beginnings of a screen addiction growing in our children. When we found our new home, we laid down new rules and embraced a new lifestyle.

We saw value in our children growing up with a lot of outdoor play and limited electronic use.

We didn't allow our children to watch TV, play video games, or use handheld devices **at all during the week**. Instead, we encouraged them to use their free time to jump on the trampoline, ride bikes to the playground, read, sew, create through arts and crafts, bake, play piano, and focus on getting homework done accurately, without distractions. We encouraged them to have friends

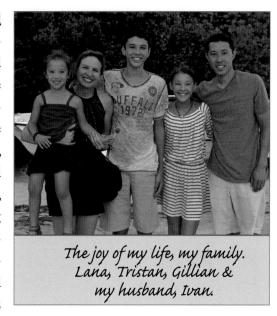

The joy of my life, my family. Lana, Tristan, Gillian & my husband, Ivan.

over. We encouraged them to have fun, without the allure of screens.

At times, we felt like the only family in town who didn't allow our kids to use electronics and our children complained about it…a lot! They were embarrassed to tell friends who were over that they couldn't play video games. One day a friend of Tristan's planned to come over but when he found out they couldn't play video games, he canceled. Tristan was inconsolable. But, we never wavered.

Years later, our decision to limit screen time was reinforced after I read the book *Irresistible: The Rise of Addictive Technology and the Business of Keeping Us Hooked* by Adam Alter, an associate professor of marketing at NYU's Stern School of Business. He begins the book with Steve Jobs unveiling the Apple iPad.

> *For ninety minutes, Jobs explained why the iPad was the best to look at photos, listen to music, take classes on iTunes, browse Facebook, play games, and navigate thousands of apps. He believed everyone should own an iPad…..But he refused to let his kids use the device.*[36]

Eventually, our children's friends got used to the idea that playdates at our home did not include a screen. Over the grammar school years, packs of boys built bamboo forts in our yard, played weekly street hockey games, Gillian's friends created elaborate choreography to the latest songs, and they all learned backflips on the trampoline. Tristan and Gillian's friends knew if they came over they were either going to break a sweat or use their brain to create. We knew we were on to something because our home was always full of children, even without access to screens. Perhaps kids actually craved this kind of play. It made us so happy to watch our children grow up with a strong sense of community and confidence. They took advantage of all our community had to offer. Then our son, Tristan, entered middle school.

DUN-DUN-DUUUUN!!!!

The big talk around town the summer before middle school revolved around when kids should get a smartphone. Some 5th graders had received one for graduation; others were getting them right before middle school started. Never one to transition smoothly to anything new, we decided to make Tristan earn a phone. He would have to maintain good grades, be responsible, and get to the bus stop on time before getting an expensive phone to call his own. As one of the few 6th graders without a phone at his middle school, Tristan was so frustrated! He struggled with not being part of text groups to make plans with friends, and felt humiliated when teachers would let kids use their phones as part of a lesson and he didn't have one. This lack of technology made him feel like an outcast and he was <u>certain</u> he was the only kid in the WORLD who was unconnected. As much as he was struggling, he got all A's the first marking period...his best report card ever! Without the distraction of social media, texting, and gaming, Tristan concentrated at school and focused on homework. It didn't hurt that we were dangling the phone like a carrot, and he was hungry.

And then it happened! By his 12th birthday, Tristan was the proud owner of his very own phone. To subsidize the cost of the phone he was walking the dog, putting away laundry, setting the table, changing his sheets, mowing the lawn, and doing yard work. If his chores didn't get done, his phone was taken away until they were. At first, he managed well having a phone. Within weeks though, we noticed a decline in all areas of Tristan's life. At first, we noted a marked decrease in friends coming over. My house once was full of boys; now Tristan gamed online with his friends in virtual reality instead of physically having them over. There were also more disagreements with everyone in the family. His relationship with his sister, Gillian, became very strained and now the littlest thing she did would set him off. After being reprimanded, he would skulk away and be moody for the rest of the day. He'd disappear and then reappear much later with glassy eyes and a zoned-out look. His grades began to decline. He withdrew from the family.

Tristan was irritable if he wasn't near his phone. We joked that his phone was his "woobie."* He could not control the urge to check his phone. If someone texted or FaceTimed him, he would have to answer them immediately. His behavior was alarming. When we noticed these behaviors, we set stricter limits and didn't let him have his phone at night. He remained edgy, irritable, and unfocused. We had moved to an outdoor-nurturing community, yet we had a child who was content to stay inside all day. Toward the end of seventh grade, there were three incidents involving electronic use that forced us to reevaluate our parenting.

*Woobie: any object, typically a blanket, garment or stuffed animal used for comfort.

Strike 1

One Saturday night, Tristan invited some friends over to play video games in his room. While there was a TV in his room, there was no cable. Several hours later, the boys came down red-faced and looking guilty. "What game were you boys playing?" No reply. "What were you doing up there?" Crickets. Finally, one boy sheepishly admitted that they had watched an R-rated movie through a friend's Netflix account. Good grief.

Strike 2

Tristan's grade in science wasn't very good, yet he seemed motivated to improve it by excelling on an upcoming test. Every night for a week he went into his room with his computer to "focus without any distractions." But when we saw his test score, it was mediocre at best. A family friend suggested that we check the history on his computer. Imagine our surprise when we discovered that Tristan had been watching episodes of a TV comedy rather than studying!

Strike 3

Banned from doing work in his room, Tristan asked if he could do his homework in the formal living room because his siblings were a distraction. I gave him permission and went back to cooking dinner. After a few minutes, I went in to check on him. While his hands were on the keyboard, his eyes were in his lap. He was watching a cartoon on his phone!

We were done.

Not only was Tristan addicted to electronics, we no longer could trust him. He had always been honest, but the desire to be in front of a screen was leading him to be sneaky in order to satisfy those desires. We needed to help him restore his good character. We signed him up to be a church altar server and gave him more responsibilities around our home. If he became too irritated by his siblings during dinner, he did the dishes. We had countless talks with him about being honest, respecting his father and me when making decisions, and what benefits are gained

Then the phone call came from the school principal.

by being completely focused on your work. We thought he was taking it all in...growing, maturing, finding balance with his phone.

Then the phone call came from the school principal.

Tristan got into trouble speaking about a classmate. The intent was innocent, but the consequence was undeniable. Tristan's words hurt another student. And now he was being reprimanded by the principal.

My husband and I sat motionless as we heard the story. We could not help but agree on the punishment; we had to take away Tristan's phone, not for a day, not for a week, but for the entire summer between 7th and 8th grade. Some parents may argue that our punishment was too harsh; others would argue it wasn't harsh enough. But we agreed to stick by our decision, no matter how difficult the circumstances would become around our home.

But, like most storms it passed, and within a week it was calm again.

At first, Tristan was totally lost without his phone. He could not text his friends and calling them from our house phone was beneath his dignity. He was disconnected from social media; how would he know what was going on with his friends? Taking away his smartphone left a tangible void in his life.

But, like most storms it passed, and within a week it was calm again. Tristan rode his bike to friends' homes rather than suffer the embarrassment of calling them from the house phone. He became more social around the house and dinner table. His sister commented, "My brother is back!" Our son had always been a happy youngster,

A LEAP OF FAITH
CHLOE'S STORY AS TOLD BY DR. D
Eighth Grader

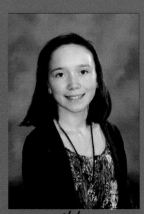

Chloe

When I met Chloe, she was 10 years old and already wearing eyeglasses. She had one of the highest prescriptions I've managed in such a young student, yet she was not the stereotypical child found among many of my younger patients who suffered from myopia. Chloe rarely entertained herself with electronics; her mother was a seasoned teacher who witnessed in her classroom the obsession that rapidly develops with handheld devices. Chloe's parents actively encouraged hobbies that stimulated independent thinking. She adores origami, enjoys needlepoint and she's an avid reader, exhibiting a vocabulary that rivals most adults. Yet, despite all efforts, Chloe's eyesight continually worsened. Her parents sought our care to address her progressively deteriorating eyesight.

I recall the consultation as if it were yesterday. Chloe and her mother were so pleased when they found out there were options to correct her vision, while possibly arresting her myopia. However, her dad was not convinced. Like so many parents, he had never heard of orthokeratology and was apprehensive, if not skeptical. After all, these were his daughter's eyes! I recall meeting with him separately and reviewing, step-by-step, how this technology works. My consultation went something like this:

 Step 1: We use the measurements taken from Chloe's eye examination to design a custom contact lens that has no corrective prescription. This is orthokeratology.

 Step 2: Chloe applies the custom-made contact lens to her eyes just prior to sleeping. Arrows show the orthokeratology lens.

 Step 3: As she sleeps, the lenses will gently reshape the front surface of her eyes (the cornea). Arrows show the newly reshaped cornea.

 Step 4: Upon waking, Chloe will remove the contact lenses.

 Step 5: Chloe's precisely re-shaped corneas will allow her to see without eyeglasses throughout the entire day.

Chloe's dad was indeed impressed, but even more conflicted. "Reshape my daughter's eyes?" He asked. "Won't that hurt? Would too much pressure be put on her eyes and cause problems later on? What if she rubs her eyes when she's sleeping?"

His questions were appropriate and his concerns valid and I patiently addressed each one. After a few days, he agreed to take a leap of faith and agree to the treatment for his daughter. Like so many parents he was torn, weighing the risk of wearing contact lenses against the increasing risk of sight-threatening problems as Chloe's prescription further deteriorated.

Orthokeratology is a treatment not to be taken lightly. A successful outcome is determined by the expertise and experience of the doctor providing it. Unlike traditional contact lenses, orthokeratology reshapes the child's eye, requiring skill and consistent follow-up to assure proper vision correction is achieved, safely and without unnecessarily exposing your child to unnecessary risk, such as infection.

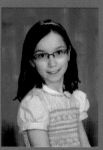

Chloe in 4th grade

In Chloe's case, the outcome could not have been better. Her dad? He's the biggest fan of the technique! Orthokeratology allowed his daughter to experience life without the limitations created by eyeglasses. Her vision has not gotten worse since she started the treatment several years ago…a welcome "side effect" after taking a leap of faith.

and now he seemed to be a happier, more content, more social, more engaged teen.

We didn't realize it at the time, but Tristan's punishment had been a gift. It was the kind of 1970s summer my husband and I enjoyed as kids. It was full of swimming, biking, hiking, going for ice cream, and enjoying independence and freedom.

We took the family on a big trip out west to visit three national parks at the end of the summer. We begrudgingly decided that Tristan could use his phone during the trip. We were worried that his old behaviors would return, but he surprised us. The summer detox was successful! Watching him with his phone had always caused us to feel uneasy and irritated, but we actually experienced joy in watching him capture images of the beautiful scenery and jam along to his favorite tunes.

But our challenges are not over...

Tristan has two younger sisters. We attempted to apply the lessons we learned with Tristan to his siblings. And it worked for the most part with our middle daughter, Gillian. But, the youngest sister, Lana Reagan, came with a new set of challenges. Unlike our older kids, Lana was brought up with accessibility to handheld electronics almost from birth. She used to marvel as her older brother would entertain himself with his computer or smartphone. Lana would want to (almost demand to) hold the device in her own hands, even as an infant.

Never a good sleeper, she began using a tablet when she was about three years old. If she slept through the night, she could earn twenty minutes on the tablet while I was cooking dinner. It worked like a charm. Now at four years old, she will often ask if I'm going to cook dinner right after breakfast! This is a child who loves the outdoors. She walks to preschool almost every day, rides a two-wheeler in cold weather, and plays soccer and ice hockey. Yet, she thinks about her screen time obsessively. We've seen firsthand with Tristan how addictive a screen can be. We don't want Lana to ever become addicted to screens but how can we ensure that she grows up with limited access to this inescapable magnet?

We will be able to shield Lana from all electronic use through grammar school, but after that it becomes nearly impossible. All students receive their very own laptop or tablet the first day of 6th grade! They use it in virtually every class, bring it home each night, and do most of their homework on it. Our child will be on a screen for more than several hours a day doing schoolwork. Presently, we see it with Gillian, our 8th grader. She spends <u>hours</u> most nights, staring at the screen completing homework and projects. Although we don't allow her to use her tablet for social media or video games, she still tallies many hours a week staring at her screen.

Screen addiction has become the most forceful, recurring obstacle in achieving and maintaining the kind of lifestyle we imagined for our family. As a young teacher, I envisioned raising well-adjusted children by continually exposing them to our core family values. What I could not foresee at the time is how insidious and relentless technology could be. It would infiltrate every aspect of our lives AND the amount of time, energy and commitment necessary to off-set its effect on my family could be overwhelming.

However, I firmly believe my goal as a mother, a teacher, a human being is achievable through focus and dedication...and it's well worth the effort!

You Set the Tone...Here's How!

Nicholas Despotidis

Raising Happy Children

There are tears in the young mother's eyes as she watches her child struggle to see the eye chart. She can't believe what is clear to her is blurry to her young child. "Isn't there anything you can do? My child's vision keeps getting worse!" Unfortunately, this scenario is not uncommon in my exam room.

Parents are often unaware of how poorly their child sees until it is illustrated in my exam room. My day centers around addressing their concerns and answering their questions. My honest and emphatic reply is simple, "Allow your child to play outside two hours a day. Every day." This elicits a dazed and confused look from most parents, as if I was speaking in Greek.

"Two hours a day? I work!"
"Alice has too much homework to get done."
"Johnny has no one to play with, what would he do?"

The goal of every parent is to raise happy and healthy kids, but we don't always know how to do that. The reality is that there is no *one* answer or *one* right plan. It's different for every child, every family.

I've had the privilege of examining thousands of children who are now adults. In my more than three decades as an eye doctor, I've learned to look beyond eyesight and evaluate the whole child. There is not a distinct line between raising children with healthy vision and raising happy children. That's because the two are related.

As a young optometrist, I felt that my role as an eye doctor was to detect and address visual anomalies, like myopia. However, as I've matured as a clinician, my role as a healthcare provider evolved to fill a void that addressed more than just a child's eyes and vision. I've witnessed children in my exam chair who excelled in school but fell short in life skills. We are all familiar with IQ or a person's *intelligence quotient*. But, there is also the EQ *(emotional quotient)* and LQ *(love quotient)*.[37] Myopia, or nearsightedness, has reached epidemic levels. I believe that is due in part to our obsession with IQ, at the cost of neglecting EQ or LQ.

Among many parents who visit my office, a drive for scholastic excellence in their children is understandable. For many of them, scholastic advancement was the gateway to a better life, a richer life, a more comfortable life. That was the case with my family, who emigrated from Europe with nothing more than hopes of a better future for their children. My parents valued education above all else; they viewed it as their children's avenue to a better life. As a result, when I came home with a 99% on a test they'd often comment, "What happened?"

Obsession with academic achievement has come at a cost. With the growing accessibility to knowledge through technology, our good intentions as parents may have yielded an unwanted result: children who are myopic visually AND socially! Activities requiring imagination, socialization, even confrontation have been replaced with screen time. We no longer value the outdoor activities that naturally develop social skills or EQ: jumping rope, riding bicycles, and dare I say, being bored!

> There is not a distinct line between raising children with healthy vision and raising happy children.

Children in my exam chair appear lonelier despite having dozens of virtual "friends." Compassion, a component many agree is critical to happiness, may be replaced with envy or the feeling of not being good enough. Face-to-face interaction is vital to developing both an emotional

> ## Obsession with academic achievement has come at a cost.

quotient and love quotient. Many of the skills that led to my own happy life such as grit, perseverance, compassion, empathy, and delayed gratification, were developed during interaction with my friends and not in the classroom.

I did not develop myopia until I entered college, when my focus transitioned from the basketball court to the classroom. That's the case with many of our parents; they either never wore eyeglasses or started wearing them later in life. Even parents with high levels of myopia have children whose eyeglass prescriptions rival their own, but at much younger ages.

Leadership, grit, and screen obsession are interconnected. In order to address the myopia epidemic among our children, I believe it requires more than simply playing outside, wearing special contact lenses, or instilling eye drops. It requires a paradigm shift from stressing scholastic overachievement to nurturing social skills. This is why, as an optometrist, I extol the importance of nurturing social skills as much, if not more than intellectual skills. Myopia does not just describe eyesight, it can describe a personality type.

Insight #1: Eye-to-Eye Contact is More Important than Visual Acuity

We need face-to-face interaction to be happy. All the accounts that I've read, from college students to centenarians, implies regular face-to-face interaction cultivates happiness in human beings. Screen-to-screen interaction does not fulfill this primal need.

I've offered workshops for students and their parents through the years, outlining steps to preserve children's eyesight. During one workshop, we aired the documentary *Screenagers: Growing Up in the Digital Age*.[38] Through it, I've learned some valuable lessons. For example, author Simon Sinek commented, "Making eye contact really, really matters. There's a reason that no one has signed a peace treaty over a video conference."

> Work on establishing activities that inspire outdoor play.

But if children are having less eye contact with their peers, how is this skill developed or enhanced? The answer is...it may NOT! Myopia may develop from too much indoor activity, but more ominously, indoor activities may keep our children from personally socializing with friends, a prerequisite for happiness.

It's a sign of the times when parents who can't attend one of my workshops requests that we videotape the lecture or air them live via the Internet. My response is always the same:

> *My entire talk is about the importance of eye-to-eye contact. It's lacking in our children's education. They play video games with friends without being in the same room! While videotaping the presentation or showing it online is convenient and easy to do, it contradicts the message that I'm committed to. Our children have enough screen time. It is causing the myopia epidemic. We will have another seminar soon and I hope you and your child can make that one. Thank you for your suggestion.*

Work on establishing activities that inspire outdoor play. Encourage friendships with your children's peers who consistently enjoy outdoor activities. We inherently enjoy when our children study with like-minded peers, but often neglect balancing our children's exposure to others who are naturally drawn to the outdoors.

Insight #2: Computers are Persuasive Technologies

"Captology" is a term I was unfamiliar with until writing this book. Captology is the study of electronics as persuasive technologies. This includes interactive devices like tablets, computers, video games, and smartphones created for the purpose of influencing our behaviors.

The following was taken from Stanford's Persuasive Technology Lab:[39]

> *The field of captology and persuasive technology is growing quickly. Every day more computing products, including websites and mobile apps, are designed to change what people think and do.*

This didn't come as a surprise. We've all experienced our subconscious and conscious preferences seeming to magically appear while viewing websites and search engines. Business empires are built on designing software with the sole intention of keeping us engaged on screens as long as possible.

Insight #3: Knowing is One Thing, Doing is Another!

When I was young, "no" meant "no." My parents' decisions were final! Unfortunately, in my case, this strategy didn't always work with my sons. Instead, researchers advocate educating our children about the <u>reason</u> for setting boundaries.[40] Explain <u>why</u> you've set limits.

After you explain to your child why you're limiting their screen time, how do you transition them off their devices? Remember, their obsession with electronics is due in part to a neurotransmitter called dopamine, which helps them associate enjoyment with electronic usage.

In the documentary *Screenagers* they recommended three steps: Dialogue, Limits, Warnings.

We've discussed the first step, *dialogue*. What about *limits*? Bring your child into the decision regarding when to stop. If they have ownership of the time limits, the greater the likelihood they'll comply when that time is reached. Some experts recommend having a timer set while kids are playing video games. I asked parents to set timers for their children who read excessively in my earlier book, *My Children Are Nearsighted Too*. Electronics have raised the threshold and it's even harder to get them to respond to an external signal. Some parents set two signals, a timer AND a snooze button, to act as a warning that time's come to an end. Regardless of your strategy:

1. The key is to discuss <u>why</u> you're setting limits
2. Agree upon how long your child will use electronics for entertainment
3. Set clear warnings with consequences, if those warnings are not followed

Keep in mind when we play computer games or interact with any electronic device, our brain's dopamine receptors are stimulated. However, our brain adapts to this continual stimulation by physically decreasing the quantity of dopamine released in our brains. More and more screen time is needed to achieve the same pleasurable feelings. For this reason, many experts recommend limiting screen time for entertainment purposes to 30-minute intervals.

> My personal recommendation from the exam chair is no more than 1 hour of electronic use for entertainment during school days, and limiting the use to 2 hours on days off.

My personal recommendation from the exam chair is no more than 1 hour of electronic use for entertainment during school days, and limiting the use to 2 hours on days off. And this includes television. TV will snatch our children's attention keeping them indoors, away from social interaction. It also leads to the number one reason children (and their parents) have trouble completing assignments on time: time management.

Insight #4: Time Management = Life Management

My son Nicholas attended one of my seminars on leadership. In that presentation, I introduced the concept of "time management." Although there were 100 students and parents in attendance, I was speaking directly to him. Like most parents, I've struggled to teach my sons how to manage their time. It's understandable; it took me my entire adulthood to achieve good organizational skills! Why would I expect my sons to acquire a skill that's so elusive to me and so many others?

EISENHOWER DECISION MATRIX

	URGENT	NOT URGENT
IMPORTANT	**1** Important and Urgent	**2** Important but NOT Urgent
NOT IMPORTANT	**3** NOT Important but Urgent	**4** NOT Important NOT Urgent

Students have trouble understanding box #3: NOT Important but Urgent.

I asked the attendees, "What stands in your way of achieving your goals?" I heard several excuses, and when I heard "procrastination," I exclaimed, "Time management!" The parents cheered with joy! The students looked like perplexed puppies with their heads tilted to the side.

One concept that's helped me explain the concept of time management is the "Eisenhower Decision Matrix."[41] It puts our activities into four categories:

1. **Do First** Important and urgent
2. **Schedule** Important but not urgent
3. **Delegate** Not important but urgent
4. **Don't Do!** Not important and not urgent

This was a new concept to a lot of the students in the room, including my son. Most felt all of their activities fell into the first category....**Important and Urgent**.

I asked for examples that fit each category:

1. *Important and urgent* The most common response was, homework that's due the next day.

2. *Important but not urgent* Some examples included, an assignment due next week, piano practice, eating, brushing their teeth. (Now they're getting it, I thought to myself...)

3. *Not important but urgent* ...crickets, silence, not one response. The concept of something being urgent but NOT important was totally foreign to the students. They felt every urgency was important, and that was the value of my lesson. After lots and lots of cajoling on my part, students began to offer up examples.

    "Like when my friend texts me a question and expects me to get back to them immediately?"

    "When a TV show is about to start and I really want to watch it?"

    "When my friend posts something online and expects me to respond to it immediately?"

Slowly, they got it. What may be important to others is not neces-sarily important to you and it may stop you from obtaining your goals or finishing an assignment.

4. *Not important and not urgent* There was no shortage of responses: television, video games, texting friends, social media sites. And then I asked them, "What category do you spend most of your time in?" It was unanimous….not important and not urgent.

Insight #5: Perfection is a Myth

"Tell Dr. D what you got on your SAT."
"1530," the student answered as she sheepishly looked over at her mother.
"Are you happy with your performance?" I asked.
"Well, my mother isn't."

I turn to the parent, not able to hide my look of befuddle-ment. Her mother sputters, "She could have done better in the verbal section!"

I'm obviously not a college advisor, but I <u>do</u> know that when we teach our

> I've learned that in order to succeed in life, we have to take chances in the face of possible failure, at the risk of not being perfect.

children to strive for perfection and let them know we will be disap-pointed with anything less, they are missing other valuable lessons. I've learned that in order to succeed in life, we have to take chances in the face of possible failure, at the risk of not being perfect. If leaders wait for perfect decisions, they will never lead. Progression and pro-motion stem from forward movement, despite mistakes, not in their absence. According to retired United States Army General Stanley McChrystal, "As a leader, you fail every day." But he follows up by saying, "Leaders can let you fail, but not let you <u>be</u> a failure!".[42]

Sensing an opportunity to help both the student and parent in front of me, I decided to tell them the story of Jack Ma, the founder of Alibaba and one of the richest men in the world. As a young man, Mr. Ma failed several entrance exams in primary and middle schools. He even failed his college entrance exams...twice! The student in front of me scored in the 99th percentile of all children taking the SAT with her, yet she clearly felt she had failed...her mother.

Better is the enemy of good.

Undaunted, I continued and told them about Angela Duckworth, the author of the book *Grit*.[43] A research psychologist at the University of Pennsylvania, she studies traits that predict success in life, not just in school. A MacArthur Fellowship (nicknamed the "genius grant") recipient, surprisingly she doesn't theorize that success in life comes from intelligence or perfect test grades. Instead, her theory is that it is the ability to pursue worthy goals for the long term, despite adversity, setbacks, or disappointments that result in success.

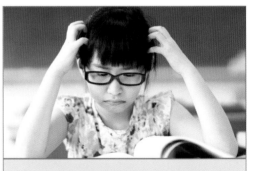

Students with very high prescriptions to correct myopia are at the highest risk for vision loss from a side effect from the condition.

My other exam rooms were filling with patients awaiting my care, but I couldn't help myself, and I continued on, "My experience is that children who are afraid to make mistakes, despite graduating from prestigious colleges, become followers rather than leaders. Better is the enemy of good."

Many of these highly driven students are the same ones who exhibit high degrees of myopia that develop at very early ages. And the two may be directly related. We refer to this high degree of myopia, over -5.00D, as "pathological." And this higher degree of nearsightedness doesn't just lead to thicker and thicker eyeglass lenses. It is also associated with a higher prevalence of vision loss due to the alteration of the shape of the eyeball. In the United States, pathological myopia is the seventh-leading cause of legal blindness.[44]

> Nurturing our children's effort, rather than the result, may go a long way to achieve our ultimate goal: happy children

In my exam chair, I see a higher prevalence of pathological myopia among ultra-driven students. A 1530 SAT score doesn't happen without dedicating yourself to this goal, often starting at a very young age.

When children develop nearsightedness under 8 years of age, they're likely to develop pathological myopia.[28] That's one reason I'm compelled to talk to parents about the ramifications of causing an imbalance for their children by applying too much academic pressure.

In my opinion, in order for pathological myopia to develop there needs to be both a genetic predisposition and an environmental demand that elicits such high degrees of myopia. I've also witnessed this high level of myopia in children whose parents don't even wear eyeglasses, demonstrating to me how much environment plays a role in its development.

I appreciate the value of striving for perfection, yet understand it does not exist. In life, as in academics, we should strive for continual improvement, not perfection. Nurturing our children's effort, rather than the result, may go a long way to achieve our ultimate goal: happy children. To address the myopia epidemic, we have to create balance in our children's lives. Balance at the expense of perfection.

INNER FULFILLMENT
GREGORY'S STORY AS TOLD BY DR. D

My wife and I were taking the 5 hour trek to see our younger son at college. Normally, we'd fill up with joy in the anticipation of seeing him. Not this time. I recall the deafening silence in the car. Gregory had called weeks earlier, distressed and unable to focus on ANYTHING but his studies. No matter how hard he tried, his focus would return to his academics. When he was out with friends, his mind would wander to the mountains of school work waiting for him back at his room. When he was at the library, his mind would drift to the sheer deprivation he was putting himself through to maintain his spot on the dean's list.

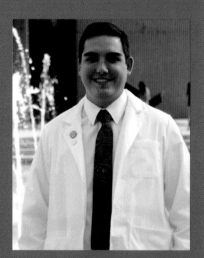

Gregory

His roommate would order Gregory to "chill," yet the monkeys in his brain continued to recite the same chant, "You're going to fail, you're not going to maintain an "A" average, you're not going to medical school!"

Every morning began by gagging and throwing up, even when there was nothing in his stomach. Finally, he sheepishly called us for help. As we drove up to his apartment, our hearts sank; our 6-foot mammoth of a son appeared emaciated, his face drawn, his eyes staring through us. We consoled him, but nothing seemed to penetrate his trance. We nervously packed his bags….no one said a word during the long journey home. We found ourselves in the waiting room of a gastroenterologist the very next day.

"We'll have to perform an endoscopy to rule things out," the physician explained.

"What kind of things?" my wife shouted.

"Ulcers…bleeding…I don't think there is something serious going on, but we have to rule everything out."

My wife turned to me, totally deflated. We scheduled the endoscopic exam for the following day.

As Gregory awaited his procedure, almost numb to all that transpired over the previous 48 hours, he recalled a conversation with the anesthesiologist just prior to sedating him. "You're pre-med? I used to throw up all the time…get used to it!" He laughed with the other physicians within earshot of his comments.

The examination revealed nothing…absolutely nothing. "Just nerves," the specialist explained. "I can prescribe some antacids, or perhaps something to calm your anxiety."

That was the last straw; my wife turned to me that night in the privacy of our home with words that will never leave me. "Stop it! Just stop it! Stop trying to make Gregory into the student you could never become! He's sick because he's expected to be an "A" student, a perfect student, and it's making him sick. I won't stand for it!"

My son, the one I'd give my life for, was sick due to my conscious and unconscious expectations. I knew my wife was right but could not help myself…until that very moment. Gregory went back to school shortly afterward and asked if he could join a fraternity. Against my better judgment, I agreed. And with that, his grades began to plummet. When I look back, I can't remember a time I was so conflicted, but my wife's words never left me.

It took Gregory four years to recover from the academic missteps after "letting go." One of those four years included obtaining a master's degree at Johns Hopkins University, obtaining a perfect 4.0 GPA, but this time there was no throwing up; just controllable, justifiable nervousness.

The difference? He grew up. His academic rigors now matched his ability to withstand those demands. He clarified his vision ON HIS OWN and was now prepared for the journey that awaited him on a path to realizing his goals.

It took the wisdom of my older son, Nicholas, to clarify it with a fable:

He told a story about a young man who was driving with the GPS on in his car. As he drove, the GPS would shout, "Recalculating! Recalculating!" because he wasn't following the map's instructions. The young man continued to drive, making one wrong turn after another, totally ignoring the advice streaming from the GPS while it obnoxiously exclaimed, "Recalculating! Recalculating! Recalculating! Recalculating!"

Finally, the young man reached his destination, after a long, protracted journey, knowing full-well he ignored the advice of the GPS. He beamed with pride because he realized his goal….and he did it on his own.

Hence the lesson: Dad = GPS

Insight #6: Sleep is Not Optional

Zzzzzzzzz...... The importance of sleep is well documented, yet children are not sleeping as much as when I started practicing 30 years ago and many are perpetually sleep deprived. Could it be because they have 24-hour access to information on the worldwide web and are online with friends throughout the night? When I was younger, studying was over when the library closed. However, with the Internet, this self-imposed deadline no longer exists.

How much sleep is enough? The National Sleep Foundation recommends 8 to 10 hours of sleep each night, yet a fraction of teens get close to this number.[45] Even though physicians agree sleep is necessary to assure proper mental and physical development, it is taken for granted. Sleep deprivation increases the likelihood teens will suffer a myriad of negative consequences, including an inability to concentrate, poor grades, anxiety, and depression.[45,46] Unfortunately, sleep deprived teens are common in my exam room. Some stare at me blankly, some break down and cry, not able to verbalize their stress, but clearly exhausted.

Orthokeratology contact lenses that I prescribe to slow down or stop myopia from progressing require at least 6 hours of sleep to be effective. Yet, even some middle school students have a hard time achieving this amount of sleep. This is why I talk about the importance of sleep to all my younger patients. But I'm fighting an uphill battle.

"The research is clear that adolescents who get enough sleep have a reduced risk of being overweight or suffering depression...and have better grades, higher standardized test scores, and an overall better quality of life," states Judith Owens, MD, MPH, Director of Sleep Medicine, and lead author of a new policy statement from the American Academy of Pediatrics on delayed start times for high school students. "Studies have shown that delaying early school start times is one key factor that can help adolescents get the sleep they need to grow and learn."[47]

A conference on adolescent sleep was the topic of a recent *New York Times* article, "The Science of Adolescent Sleep," by Perri Klass, MD.[48] The article reported that later school start times are advocated to help teens get the sleep their body requires for proper physical and mental development. In the article, Charles Czeisler, PhD, MD, a professor of sleep medicine at Harvard Medical School, was quoted as saying:

> *The brain needs sleep to replenish energy sources....Sleep is critical to maintain focus and alertness, to repair and maintain brain cells, to clear out toxic metabolites.*

Teenagers also struggle to get out of bed in the morning and recent research provides insight into why.[49] The teen's biological clock seems to shift forward during puberty, making youngsters want to go to sleep later and wake up later. This sleep delay is common and tends to disappear in the late teens.

Melatonin is a hormone produced in the brain that triggers sleepiness.[50] The blue light emitted from screens on tablets and smartphones have been shown to reduce melatonin secretion in the brain, further delaying when teens feel sleepy.[51] The cognitive stimulation just prior to bedtime can also be a factor. For these reasons, I recommend all my student patients avoid ALL electronics one hour prior to sleeping. If the student must study, they should read a textbook or flash cards, but do not use a computer or other electronic device.

I recall one newsletter to parents, educating them on the effects electronics, specifically blue light, may have on their children's sleep. Within minutes of the email going out, a parent rebutted, "There are

> I recommend all my student patients avoid ALL electronics one hour prior to sleeping.

apps and screens that block blue light!" I had to think long and hard before responding to this somewhat defensive parent.

I'm aware phone and other manufactures have developed "blue light" filters to lessen the possible adverse effect of looking at electronics before bed. But there are no studies that I'm aware of that have demonstrated blue filters, at very dim intensities, are effective in preventing the disruption caused by light exposure at night. And besides, shutting down electronics gives our children an opportunity to disconnect and to decompress from their day.

Whether the answer is later school start times or turning off electronics 60 minutes prior to sleeping, parents have to take an active role in ensuring their children are obtaining at least 8 hours of sleep per night. Parents tell me the best way to accomplish this goal is imposing realistic deadlines for completing homework and removing the smartphone from their children's rooms. And the number one excuse given for not following through on my recommendation? "I use my phone as an alarm clock." To which I respond, with an empathetic grin, "Dust off your old alarm clock and leave your phone outside the bedroom."

Insight #7: Successful Multitasking is a Myth

Kids pride themselves on their ability to instant message, complete homework assignments, and respond to text messages all while listening to music or watching videos online. However, successful multitasking is a myth. Studies show instead that trying to do more than one thing at a time reduces our efficiency since it takes longer to complete each task.[52]

Children demand so much from themselves. There is peer pressure to do well. The homework load is daunting. And when the student needs a break, they have plenty of distractions online. Many parents are unaware of how much verbal (and non-verbal) pressure they put on their children. I know when my sons brought home a "B," I often wondered to myself, "Did they work hard enough?" Even if I didn't say it out loud, my sons knew my expectations and probably could sense my disappointment.

Insight #8: Don't Do What I Do, Do What I Say

"Dad, take your own advice and put your phone down! What would your patients say?" Yes, like most people, I have trouble putting down my phone. Yet, it disturbs me when I see families out, absorbed in some virtual world instead of enjoying the real world around them. I've given and heard every excuse:

"I had an urgent message."

"I'm a moderator for a parents association, sports team, etc."

"I'm working from home."

"I have to check the weather, traffic, reviews, etc."

The reality is that children respond to what we do, not what we say, and that's the truth. When it comes to helping your child, knowing what to do and doing it are two different things.

> The reality is that children respond to what we do, not what we say, and that's the truth.

So, like you, I'm human and I make mistakes...many mistakes. But, I try to learn from them and would like to share these four tips with both parents and patients:

1. Schedule periods to leave your phone at home to assure you're not tempted to find an excuse to pick it up
2. No electronics at the dinner table
3. No electronics in the bedroom
4. No phone where you do your most cognitively demanding work (e.g., school and office work)

That's it! Four steps I preach to all my patients. If you choose to follow them, I believe your children will do the same. People (including your children) might hear what you <u>say</u>, but they always remember what you <u>do</u>.

The guide to raising children with healthy vision is deceivingly simple: balance in all things. Allow your kids to play outside, socialize with like-minded friends, and limit their access to technology, which is insidious, grabs their attention, and may be intentionally designed to be habit-forming.

The visual myopia epidemic is representative of a much deeper concern than nearsightedness among children. It is the development of social myopia produced by excessive time spent isolated with alluring technology.

Superficially it makes sense; provide support to your child and they should develop the skills to be the best they can be by getting into a superior college. The assumption being upon graduation, they'll attain a well-paying job that will lead to their ultimate happiness.

> Expect the best, demand the best, but support the effort, not the outcome.

However, the lesson learned is a narrow focus solely on academics, leaves our kids unbalanced, stressed, sleepless, and unhappy. The key to addressing the myopia epidemic is working on ourselves (parents, that means you) to have faith in our children to develop into their best selves. Expect the best, demand the best, but support the effort, not the outcome.

It's My Battle, Too

If you speak to my sons they'll quickly admit I'm a tiger dad. I talk a good talk but walk a totally different one. I can't help myself. When both my sons attended Johns Hopkins graduate programs, I was prouder than when they attended undergraduate colleges of lesser reputation for scholastic demand. And that's why I've devoted the final words in this book to things I know I should do…and work to do…but still battle to do daily. I'm proud to say I've evolved, I've learned, and I want to share my experience, including my deep intention to do the best possible for the children I'd give my life for.

In the age of "tiger moms"* and "helicopter parenting,"** myopia is just a symptom; the ultimate result of our innate desire to raise exceptional academicians at the expense of nurturing their other talents. What I've learned, however, is the effort has run amok, detracting from what every parent wants…happy children. We associate happiness with academic achievement, leading to career security. However, security is not achieved with academic achievement, and neither is happiness nor inner fulfillment.

Could it be that happiness stems from achieving self-imposed goals and actualizing them the old-fashioned way: through grit, hard work, and mistakes…not perfection? The key for our children may be just that, "self-imposed" versus "parent-imposed" goals.

It takes courage, willpower, and common sense not to get caught up in the tsunami of advice given by friends (and authors), fueling a parent's desire to expect more for and from their child. Keep in mind the goal is not high achievers, but a healthy child, in every sense of the word.

---

*Tiger Mom/Dad: the term popularized by author Amy Chua, in her bestselling parent memoir, Battle Hymn of the Tiger Mother, to describe a demanding style of parenting. Chua identified the trait as being especially common among parents of Chinese ancestry.

**Helicopter Parent: a parent who takes an overprotective or excessive interest in the life of their child or children.

Clearing Up Eye Terms

—————————— Appendix A ——————————

AAOMC — *The American Academy of Orthokeratology and Myopia Control (AAOMC)* is an organization committed to educating the general public and eye doctors about nearsightedness. Since the field of **myopia control** is still in its infancy, this organization's efforts go a long way in helping educate patients and give guidance when attempting to locate an experienced practitioner. For more information visit www.orthokacademy.com.

Accommodation — This is the term used to describe our focusing ability when looking at close objects or reading. Children normally have much greater focusing ability than adults. That's why adults often need **bifocals** or reading glasses after the age of forty.

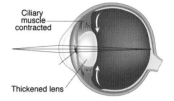

Accommodative Insufficiency — Accommodative insufficiency (AI) is a condition in which it is difficult for an individual to maintain the focus of their eyes during near tasks. This often results in blurry vision. While reading or looking at print, vision may go in and out of focus, and may be accompanied by double vision, eyestrain, or headaches. Treatments for this condition include wearing plus lenses while reading and optometric **vision therapy**.

Amblyopia — Also known as "lazy eye," amblyopia is a condition in which the **visual cortex** in the brain fails to mature properly resulting in reduced vision in an otherwise healthy eye. It can be caused by an eye turn (**strabismus**), significant degrees of uncorrected or unequal refractive error, or any condition that causes deprivation of vision in early life. Sometimes a lazy eye can be

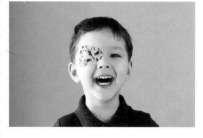

improved with glasses alone, however more severe cases may require patching or **atropine**, in order to strengthen the poorer seeing eye.

Astigmatism — When light rays don't come to a single focus, but instead focus in more than one spot (making our vision blurry at all distances), eyeglasses and contact lenses are needed that have two different powers in them. Even though it might sound scary, astigmatism is a very common eye condition!

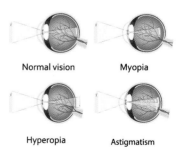

Atropine — Atropine is a medication that comes in an eye drop formulation. Eye doctors use 1% atropine eye drops to safely dilate pupils during eye examinations. Recent scientific studies have found that when very diluted (i.e. 0.01%), atropine can slow down the progression of myopia when applied nightly.

Behavioral Optometry — "Functional optometry" is another name for behavioral optometry. This is an expanded area of optometry that uses a holistic approach in the treatment of vision. **Optometrists** who pursue this type of practice are interested in how vision impacts children's daily lives. They undertake post-doctoral certification in the College of Optometrists in Vision Development (**COVD**).

Bifocal – Bifocals are eyeglasses or contact lenses that have two separate powers; the top normally for distance and the bottom normally for near. They are made in several variations, many of which eliminate the appearance of the line differentiating the two powers. In our book, we've discussed the use of bifocals in a select group of children, in an effort to slow down their **myopia** (**nearsightedness**) progression.

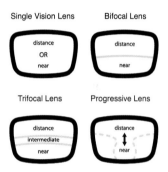

Captology — Captology is the study of computers as persuasive technologies. This includes the design, research, ethics and analysis of interactive computing products (computers, mobile phones, websites, wireless technologies, mobile applications, video games, etc.) created for the purpose of changing people's attitudes or behaviors. BJ Fogg derived the term "captology" in 1996 from an acronym: Computers As Persuasive Technologies = CAPT.

Cataract — A cataract is a clouding of the **crystalline lens** found inside the eye. Since cataracts are a normal part of aging, everyone will develop cataracts! However, cataracts have been reported at earlier ages among people with high degrees of **myopia** (**nearsightedness**).

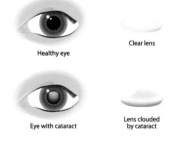

Circadian Rhythm — The circadian rhythm is the body's natural cycle of sleep/wake patterns, occurring once every 24 hours in humans. This biological process is regulated by **melatonin**, the hormone that makes us feel drowsy at night. Melatonin levels rise in the evening, peak overnight, and drop in the early morning. Blue light given off from electronic screens has been shown to inhibit melatonin and disrupt sleep cycles.

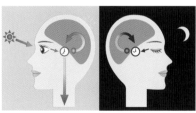

Convergence Excess — Convergence excess is the term used to describe an eye muscle imbalance that causes a tendency for the eyes to aim more inwardly than needed, usually during near work. This may result in double vision, or symptoms of eyestrain, headaches, and intermittent blurry vision. Individuals may suffer academically or avoid near tasks, and are more prone to motion sickness and dizziness. The treatment for this condition often includes a combination of glasses and **vision therapy**.

Convergence Insufficiency — Convergence insufficiency is a common near vision problem affecting children. In contrast to **convergence excess**, children with convergence insufficiency have a tendency for their eyes to drift outward during near work. This results in double vision, eyestrain, headaches, blurred vision, sleepiness, difficulty concentrating, a feeling of print moving while reading, and loss of comprehension after short periods of reading. **Vision therapy** and/or prism glasses are often required to treat this condition.

COVD — COVD stands for College of Optometrists in Vision Development. Fellows of the College (**FCOVD**) have certified their competency in this area and often refer to themselves as **behavioral or functional optometrists**. For more information visit www.COVD.org.

Cornea — The clear outer portion of the eye is called the cornea. This is the part of the eye that is first responsible for bending light rays when they enter the optical system. The cornea is also the part of the eye that contact lenses rest on and is *temporarily* reshaped with **corneal reshaping** contact lenses.

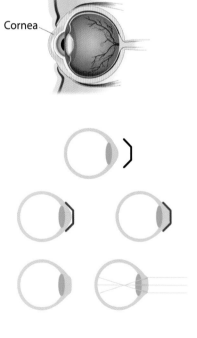

Corneal Reshaping — Also referred to as orthokeratology, Ortho-k, OK lens, Corneal Refractive Therapy (CRT®) and Vision Shaping Treatment (VST™), corneal reshaping describes the use of specially designed contact lenses, used only at night, to correct **nearsightedness** (**myopia**) during the daytime. The technique is totally reversible unlike **LASIK** or corneal refractive surgery, which makes it ideal for children who do not want to wear eyeglasses. In addition, studies indicate children who wear corneal reshaping lenses do not progress in myopia as rapidly as kids wearing daytime contact lenses or eyeglasses.

Corneal Topography — A corneal topographer is a computer driven instrument that accurately measures the very front surface of the eye (**cornea**), in order to properly fit contacts and **corneal reshaping** lenses. Not all eye doctors have this instrument in their office.

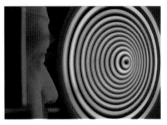

Crystalline Lens — The lens inside the eye that focuses light rays is called the crystalline lens. The crystalline lens is the structure of the eye that is responsible for changing focus so we can see objects both up close and far away, or **accommodate**. When there is a lack of transparency or cloudiness in the crystalline lens it is called a **cataract**.

Diopter — A diopter is the unit of measurement signifying the optical power of a lens. The higher the dioptric power of a lens, the more light rays are refracted. Diopters are typically divided into 0.25D steps.

Dopamine — Dopamine is a neurotransmitter found in the body with many functions, playing a major role in reward-motivated behavior. Most types of rewards increase dopamine levels in the brain. Researchers now believe that dopamine in the **retina** may regulate the development of **nearsightedness** by inhibiting connective tissue growth in the **sclera**. This translates into less eye growth over time, or less nearsightedness.

EQ (Emotional Quotient) — Emotional intelligence or emotional quotient is the capability of individuals to recognize their own emotions and those of others, discern between different feelings and label them appropriately, use emotional information to guide thinking and behavior, and manage and/or adjust emotions to adapt to environments or achieve one's goal(s).

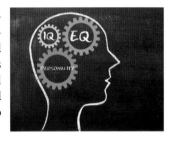

Esophoria — As our children read, we assume their eyes are working together as a team, allowing them to scan across the page efficiently. This is not always the case. When our children's eyes have a tendency to over converge or point inward, eye doctors refer to this eye teaming problem as esophoria. There are different degrees of esophoria, which can be addressed with **bifocals** or **vision therapy**.

Exophoria — In contrast to **esophoria**, children with exophoria have a tendency for their eyes to point outward. Some children with moderate to high exophoria experience eye teaming issues as well. These children display convergence problems such as **convergence insufficiency**, impairing their ability to read efficiently. This condition is treated with in-office **vision therapy**.

Farsightedness — When a person's eyes can focus more clearly on objects far away than objects up close, it is called farsightedness or **hyperopia**.

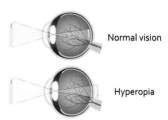

Normal vision

Hyperopia

FAAO – You may notice letters after your doctor's credentials, yet may not have an idea what they stand for. A fellow of the American Academy of Optometry (FAAO) is a voluntary post-doctoral certification for **optometrists** and other health professionals who are committed to professional vision care through lifelong learning. Fellows of the American Academy of Optometry demonstrate their knowledge and professionalism by submitting unique cases and passing an oral examination.

FCOVD — The College of Optometrists in Vision Development (COVD) is a non-profit, international membership association of eye care professionals including **optometrists**, optometry students, and vision therapists. Their primary aim is to drive progress through clinical excellence and research in developmental vision care, optometric **vision therapy**, and rehabilitation. Optometrists who successfully complete their certification process are Board Certified in Vision Development and Vision Therapy and are designated fellows of COVD (FCOVD).

FIAOMC — The International Academy of Orthokeratology and Myopia Control (IAO) is a non-profit, independent organization and represents **orthokeratology** and myopia control around the world. A fellow (FIAOMC) is someone whom the Academy has recognized as having made a significant contribution to the practice of orthokeratology. This prestigious award is an acknowledgment of commitment to the profession, experience and accomplishments.

Fovea — The fovea is a part of the eye located in the center of the **macula** region of the **retina** and is where our clearest, central vision takes place.

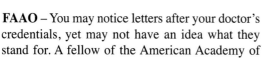

Glaucoma — Glaucoma is a disease where high pressure within the eye causes damage to the **optic nerve**, the nerve leading from the eye to the brain. Glaucoma is treatable with a daily regimen of eye drops, but if left untreated it will eventually cause blindness. Glaucoma is painless and does not have visual symptoms in its early stages, so it must be detected by an eye doctor. People with high degrees of

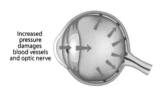

Increased pressure damages blood vessels and optic nerve

myopia (**nearsightedness**) are known to have a higher incidence of glaucoma than the general population. Other characteristics that increase the risk of glaucoma are a positive family history, age, African American or Asian heritage, diabetes, and high blood pressure.

Hyperopia — Hyperopia is another term for **farsightedness**. When a person can focus on objects far away and has trouble seeing objects up close, they are hyperopic or farsighted.

Hyperopic Defocus — Hyperopic defocus is the condition where the peripheral vision is focused behind the eye's light receptors in the **retina**, despite central vision being in focus. It has been shown that eyes with peripheral hyperopic defocus develop higher rates of **nearsightedness** than those with **myopic defocus** (defocus in front of the retina).

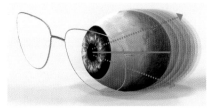

IQ (Intelligence Quotient) — The intelligence quotient (IQ) is a number representing a person's reasoning ability or intelligence, measured using problem-solving tests, as compared to the average for their age.

Iris — The colored part of the eye is the iris. When you refer to someone's eye color, you are really referring to their iris color. Even more importantly than providing a physical trait, the iris contains muscles that allow the **pupil** to get larger and allow in more light; or get smaller and restrict light.

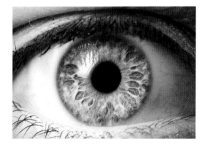

LASIK — Also known as corneal refractive surgery, LASIK stands for Laser-Assisted in Situ Keratomileusis, a complicated way of saying laser eye surgery! LASIK corrects **nearsightedness** by permanently changing the very outer layer of the **cornea**. LASIK is approved for patients over the age of 18, although we recommend waiting until after completion of academic studies before considering it. As with all surgeries, we strongly recommend investigation before undergoing LASIK. A great starting place is the FDA website, http://www.fda.gov.

LQ (Love Quotient) – A term attributed to Alibaba Group CEO Jack Ma, LQ describes a prerequisite to good leadership. The Love Quotient or LQ is something machines never have. "A machine does not have a heart, a machine does not have a soul, and a machine does not have a belief. Human beings have the souls, have

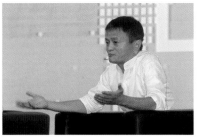

Editorial credit: SL Chen / Shutterstock.com

the belief, have the value; we are creative, we are showing that we can control the machines."

M.Ed. — The Master of Education (M.Ed. or Ed.M.; Latin Magister Educationis or Educationis Magister) is a master's degree awarded by universities in many countries. This degree in education often includes the following majors: curriculum and instruction, counseling, school psychology, and administration. It is often conferred for educators advancing in their field.

Macula — When visual acuity is discussed, we are really talking about the sharpness of focus on the back of the **retina** called the macula region. Within the macula is the **fovea**, which is responsible for clear, central vision.

Macular Degeneration — Macular degeneration is the deterioration of the **macula**, the area of the retina that is responsible for central vision. Degeneration of the macula often leads to vision loss. The likelihood of macular degeneration occurring increases with age and is also associated with high degrees of **myopia**.

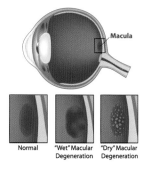

Melatonin — Melatonin is a hormone made by the pineal gland, a small gland in the brain. While it has many functions, it is the chief hormone that regulates sleep and wake cycles. Melatonin levels increase in the mid to late evening making us drowsy, and drop in the early morning hours. Melatonin levels are affected by natural light, but also tend to be affected by light given off from electronic screens. For this reason, using technology before bed may disrupt melatonin production and interfere with normal sleep cycles.

Multifocal — Multifocal refers to contact lenses that focus light across multiple distances, which were originally designed for help with near tasks in middle-aged adults. These lenses incorporate many prescriptions, focusing light at near, intermediate, and far distances. They have been shown to be effective at curtailing the progression of **nearsightedness**.

Myopia — Myopia is a vision problem where we can see clearly up close without eyeglasses, but blurry far away, hence the term **nearsightedness**. Myopia can be corrected with eyeglasses, contact lenses, **corneal reshaping**, and **corneal refractive surgery**.

Nearsightedness — The common term for **myopia** is nearsightedness. When a person has blurry vision at a distance but clear vision or sight at near, they are said to be nearsighted. A person may have nearsightedness in one or both eyes, with or without **astigmatism**.

Normal vision

Myopia

Off-label — Medications are approved by the FDA to treat specific conditions. When a medication is used for a purpose other than that approved by the FDA, it is considered an off-label use. For instance, **corneal reshaping lenses** are approved for the correction of **nearsightedness**, however they are not approved as a device to slow nearsighted progression, despite sufficient evidence supporting this use. As a result, using corneal reshaping lenses to stabilize the prescription is considered a safe, but off-label use.

Ophthalmologist — An ophthalmologist is a medical doctor (MD) who performs eye surgeries, like **LASIK**. They also diagnose and treat eye infections, prescribe eyeglasses and contact lenses. There are several subspecialties within ophthalmology. Pediatric ophthalmologists are especially important when a child has a problem requiring eye surgery.

Optic nerve — The optic nerve, also known as cranial nerve II, is the nerve that transmits visual information from the **retina** to the brain, including brightness perception, color perception and contrast (**visual acuity**). **Glaucoma** is the most common disease affecting the optic nerve, resulting in gradual, painless, loss of vision if left untreated. Individuals with higher degrees of **myopia** (**nearsightedness**) are at more risk for glaucoma than the general population.

Optician — An optician normally works with **ophthalmologists** or **optometrists** by filling eyeglass prescriptions and fitting eyewear. Some opticians are certified to fit contact lenses, but normally do not perform eye examinations.

Optometrist – Optometrists are doctors of optometry (OD), and are the main providers of vision care. They perform eye examinations, diagnose and treat vision problems and eye diseases. Drs. Despotidis and Tannen are optometrists.

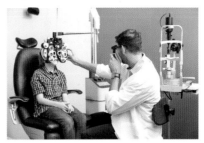

*Note from authors: Throughout the book we've referred to your child's eye professional as "eye doctor." There is understandably confusion among our patients, since there is more than one provider of vision care. Most often, **optometrists**, **opticians** and*

ophthalmologists are all involved in our children's care at one time or another. Which one is best? They're all different, yet play an important role in maintaining our children's clear eyesight. We recommend staying with the eye professional who comprehensively treats your child (and you) with respect and professionalism. Let your instinct be your guide, not the eye professional's degree, insurance plan participation or their office location. In our office we will work with all three types of eye professionals, since each fulfills specific needs for our patients.

Orthokeratology — The term used to describe the temporary improvement of **nearsightedness** with the use of specially fit contact lenses. The modern day term used to describe this technique is **corneal reshaping**.

Photoreceptors — Photoreceptors are a type of specialized sensory cells located in the **retina**. They respond to light and convert light signals into vision. Photoreceptors can be divided into two broad categories, rods and cones. Rods are important in low light level conditions and make up the majority of our peripheral vision. Cones are more sensitive in bright light conditions and make up our central and color vision.

Presbyopia — Presbyopia is a natural part of the aging process, affecting middle-aged adults and older. It occurs as the **crystalline lens** of the eye hardens and loses the ability to change shape or accommodate over time. This results in the worsening ability to focus clearly on 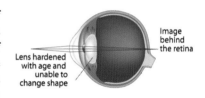 near objects and has the potential to cause headaches and eyestrain if uncorrected. This condition is treated with reading glasses or a near power addition incorporated into distance correction.

Pupil — The entrance by which light and other images enter our eyes is called the pupil. It appears as a black hole surrounded by the colored **iris** right in the middle of the eye. The pupil changes size depending on the surrounding light. In bright light it gets smaller and in dim light it gets larger.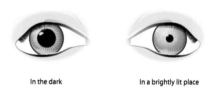

In the dark   In a brightly lit place

Retina — The retina is in the back of the eye, where images are received. This thin layer acts like a camera film capturing the picture of what we're looking at before sending it to the brain where the image is interpreted and our perception of the world is created.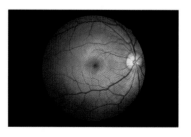

Retinal Detachment — A retinal detachment describes the condition where the **retina** pulls away from the inside of the eye. Retinal detachments are painless and may start very small but spread quickly leading to loss of vision. When a person has a retinal detachment, they will notice an increase of floaters in their vision, flashes of light, and may even notice a curtain or veil obstructing a portion of their vision. Because retinal detachments can lead to permanent vision loss, if you suspect you or someone you know has a retinal detachment, they should be seen by an eye doctor as soon as possible. Retinal detachments are more likely to occur in **nearsighted** people, especially those with higher degrees of **myopia**.

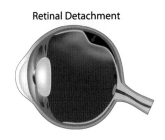

Retinal Detachment

Sclera — The visible, white part of the eyes is the sclera. It is made of strong connective tissue and helps to maintain the shape of the eyes. When our children's eyesight changes shape, the sclera is the outer layer of the eye that elongates.

Strabismus — Strabismus is a condition in which the eyes do not properly align with each other when looking at an object. If present during a large part of childhood, it may result in **amblyopia** or loss of depth perception. If onset is during adulthood, it is more likely to result in double vision. Strabismus can occur due to muscle dysfunction, **farsightedness**, problems in the brain, trauma, or infections. Types of strabismus include esotropia where the eyes are crossed; exotropia where the eyes diverge; and hypertropia where they are vertically misaligned. Treatment depends on the type of strabismus and the underlying cause. This may include the use of glasses and possibly surgery.

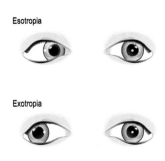

Esotropia

Exotropia

Vision Therapy — Vision therapy is also referred to as vision training and is a specialized area of optometry devoted to enhancing vision. Vision therapy trains the entire visual system, which includes eyes, brain and body. The goal of vision therapy is to train the patient's brain to use the eyes to receive information efficiently, interpret the information properly and of course react to what they see. Vision therapy is primarily practiced by a select group of doctors referred to as **behavioral optometrists**.

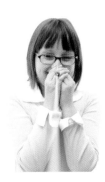

Visual Acuity — Visual acuity is the term most often used to describe the clarity of our vision. 20/20 vision refers to how clearly we see small black letters at a distance of 20 feet. The larger the denominator, the larger the letters need to be for a person to see them. So a person who has 20/70 vision needs the eye chart letters larger than the person who sees 20/20. The metric equivalent to 20/20 vision is 6/6 vision where the distance is in meters rather than feet. 20/20 vision is normally associated with "perfect" vision, however it's only an indication of how well we see at a distance.

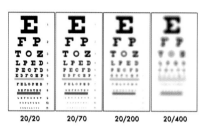

20/20   20/70   20/200   20/400

Visual cortex — The visual cortex of the brain is a part of the cerebral cortex that processes visual information. It is located in the occipital lobe in the back of the head. In **amblyopia**, parts of the visual cortex fail to develop resulting in reduced vision or poor depth perception.

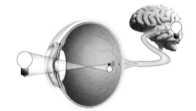

How to Read an Eyeglass Prescription:

	Sphere	Cylinder	Axis
Right Eye (OD)	-3.00	-1.00	180
Left Eye (OS)	-1.00	-2.00	180

The **sphere** component indicates the amount of **myopia (nearsightedness)** or **hyperopia (farsightedness)** present. When a negative (-) sign is in front of the number it is myopia. When a positive (+) sign is in front of the number it is hyperopia. The higher the sphere number, the greater the amount of myopia or hyperopia.

The **cylinder** component indicates the degree of **astigmatism**. This number may be positive or negative, but in either case the higher the number the greater the amount of astigmatism, or how irregularly the eye bends light. The cylinder component requires an **axis** to show how the astigmatism is lined up in the eye.

Visual Hygiene
Tips for Parents

——————— Appendix B ———————

Visual Hygiene

We've spent much of this book discussing the importance of outdoor play in raising children with healthy eyes. In this appendix, we provide additional recommendations to promote healthy visual habits.

Hold Reading Material at Least 14 Inches Away

The closer a child holds a book, the harder the eyes have to focus to maintain a clear image. Encourage your child to keep reading material, the computer monitor, handheld games, or any near work at least fourteen inches away. If your child continues to move his or her head closer and closer to the material, this may be a sign of a vision problem. There are many vision issues that would cause a child to move a book closer to his or her eyes. If you notice this behavior with your child, we'd encourage you and your child to visit an eye doctor who emphasizes a behavioral approach to eye examinations. The College of Optometrists in Vision Development certifies professional competency in this approach. You can visit www.COVD.org for more information and to find an eye doctor in your area.

Rest Every 30 Minutes

If a child reads a book, works on a computer, or plays video games for hours at a time, it can potentially cause vision problems. We encourage children to stop a near task every 30 minutes. Get up and move! Having children break from the near activity and walk around gives vision a break, too. I know, this is easier said than done. Children can be so engrossed in reading, playing a video game, or working on the computer that it can take considerable effort to even get their attention. We recommend setting a timer to act as an alarm. If it's in the same room as the child but on the other side, the simple task of checking how much time remains will get them to change to a distance focus.

Use Good Posture While Reading

We feel proper posture is critical to maintaining good vision. Proper posture allows our children to maintain an appropriate distance from their reading material. This element of posture can sometimes be overlooked, but we feel it's very important. When we examine children who have very different prescriptions between their two eyes, we'll often discover that they've developed a habit of reading or writing with their head tilted.

While it's hard to say if the head tilt occurs because of the difference in the two eyes, or the head tilt caused the difference in prescriptions, it's wise to have your child practice good posture and proper reading distance.

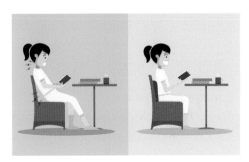

Here are some tips to avoid eye strain:

• Make sure both feet touch the floor. If your child's feet can't reach the floor, have him sit in a smaller chair or place something beneath his feet.

• The reading material should be tilted back at a 20-degree angle.

• Watch for rolled shoulders! Make sure the child is sitting upright in the chair.

• Place reading material directly in front, not off to the side. This is especially important when viewing a computer monitor.

• Ask that your child not read in bed. This is because the distance from the material to the eyes isn't controlled. When children read in bed, their posture may be distorted.

• For the same reasons mentioned above, make sure your child does not tilt his head or rest it on the desk when he reads or does near work. If your child continues to tilt his head when he is reading, even if you've corrected him many times, schedule a visit with the eye doctor.

• Light the space. We recommend an adjustable 60-watt incandescent soft white lamp or LED equivalent and avoid any source of glare on the reading material.

Atropine Drops

Appendix C

Atropine Drops

Below are questions frequently asked about
atropine therapy to prevent myopia progression

1. What is atropine?

In the past, eye doctors used 1% atropine eye drops to safely dilate children's pupils during eye examinations. More recently, it's used to treat childhood eye conditions such as lazy eye. Recent scientific studies have found that when very diluted (ie: 0.01%), atropine can slow down the progression of myopia when applied nightly.

2. Is it new?

Atropine eye drops have been used to dilate eyes for decades, however it is not FDA approved to treat myopia progression. So even though studies have found it very effective in stopping eyesight from getting worse, it is not approved for this usage.

3. Is the effect permanent?

Studies show that this treatment slows down a child's myopia degeneration for 1-2 years. Afterward, the myopia may progress rapidly. We use this drop when children are too immature to wear orthokeratology contact lenses. The diluted atropine drops buy the parents and doctors time, but it is not a permanent solution.

4. Can any doctor prescribe this eye drop and how do we get it filled?

Any doctor interested in myopia stabilization may prescribe this drop in its diluted form. The drops must be diluted from the full strength by a compound pharmacist, licensed to perform this in a sterile environment. Pharmacy compounding is an established tradition that allows a physician to prescribe a very specific medication, prepared by a pharmacist, for a patient's individual needs.

5. Is it covered by insurance?

Currently, diluted atropine drops are often not covered by prescription drug plans.

How to Choose
The Right Eye Doctor

———————— Appendix D ——————

Things to Consider When
Choosing Your Child's Eye Doctor

Is there a difference among doctors offering orthokeratology or corneal reshaping to their patients? Absolutely! As with all health-care professionals, the results achieved are based on experience, communication skills, and expertise. So how do you find the best eye doctor for YOUR child?

While many clinicians employ contact lenses to stop or slow my-opia, some use generic contact lenses designed with a "cookbook" approach to fitting children. This method may be easier to perform, but generic lenses may not take into account the individual charac-teristics of your child's eye. This can result in suboptimal vision correction or even problems. Each cornea is unique, like a finger-print, and has distinct variations in surface curvature. We can measure these variations using a machine known as a corneal topographer, which provides an elevation map of the front surface of the eye. While it is not mandatory to utilize a corneal topogra-pher in the U.S. to fit corneal reshaping lenses, we feel strongly that this instrument is necessary to properly fit these lenses.

Since most patients are children, this is critical because these young ones often cannot articulate the quality of their vision. So, results are dependent on the skill and expertise of the doctor providing the treatment.

When done correctly, orthokeratology is extremely safe. However, when this isn't the case, the results can be poor. Long-term success of treatment requires a combination of proper lens fitting, rigorous compliance to the lens care regimen, good adherence to routine fol-low-ups, and timely treatment of complications.

Having said all of the above, when enrolling your child in a myopia control program, it's the doctor who you're entrusting your children's eyesight to, not the type of lens used to correct their vision.

The CDC provides safety warning that we like to share with our patients: "Microbial keratitis is an infection of the cornea...that can cause vision loss or blindness. Improper contact lens wear, particularly poor storage case hygiene, infrequent storage case replacement, and overnight lens wear, is the largest risk factor."

Additional information about healthy contact lens wear and care is available at http://www.cdc.gov/contact lenses.

Bibliography

Appendix E

1. Dolgin E. Myopia Boom. Nature. 2015;519(7543):276-278.

2. Vitale S, Sperduto RD, Ferris FL 3rd. Increased Prevalence of Myopia in the United States Between 1971-1972 and 1999-2004. Arch Ophthalmol. 2009;127(12):1632-1639.

3. Holden BA, Fricke TR, Wilson DA, et al. Global Prevalence of Myopia and High Myopia and Temporal Trends from 2000 through 2050. Ophthalmology. 2016;123(5):1036-1042.

4. Ackland P. The Accomplishments of the Global Initiative VISION 2020: The Right to Sight and the Focus for the Next 8 Years of the Campaign. Indian J Ophthalmol. 2012;60(5):380-386.

5. Schaeffel F, Feldkaemper M. Animal Models in Myopia Research. Clin Exp Optom. 2015;98(6):507-517.

6. Pacella R, McLellan J, Grice K, Del Bono EA, Wiggs JL, Gwiazda JE. Role of Genetic Factors in the Etiology of Juvenile-Onset Myopia on a Longitudinal Study of Refractive Error. Optom Vis Sci. 1999;76(6):381-386.

7. Ramdass S, Despotidis N, Rosen CM, et al. Contact Lens Spectrum - A Retrospective Look at Children Fit with Ortho-k Lenses. Contact Lens Spectrum. 2016;31(October 2016):38-42.

8. Saw S-M, Gazzard G, Shih-Yen EC, Chua W-H. Myopia and Associated Pathological Complications. Ophthalmic Physiol Opt. 2005;25(5):381-391.

9. Read SA, Collins MJ, Vincent SJ. Light Exposure and Eye Growth in Childhood Light Exposure and Eye Growth in Childhood. Invest Ophthalmol. 2015;56(October 2015):6779-6787.

10. Cordain L, Eaton SB, Brand Miller J. An Evolutionary Analysis of the Aetiology and Pathogenesis of Juvenile-Onset Myopia. Acta. 2002;80(April 2002):125-135.

11. Young FA, Leary GA, Baldwin WR, et al. The Transmission of Refractive Errors within Eskimo Families. Am J Optom Arch Am Acad Optom. 1969;46(9):676-685.

12. Goldschmidt E. On the Etiology of Myopia. An Epidemiological Study. Acta Ophthalmol. 1968:Suppl 98:1+.

13. Rose KA, Morgan IG, Ip J, et al. Outdoor Activity Reduces the Prevalence of Myopia in Children. Ophthalmology. 2008;115(8):1279-1285.

14. Rose KA, Morgan IG, Smith W, Burlutsky G, Mitchell P, Saw S-M. Myopia, Lifestyle, and Schooling in Students of Chinese Ethnicity. Arch Ophthalmol. 2008;126(4):527-530.

15. Zhang Y, Wildsoet CF. Chapter Thirteen - RPE and Choroid Mechanisms Underlying Ocular Growth and Myopia. In: Hejtmancik JF, Nickerson JM, eds. Progress in Molecular Biology and Translational Science. Vol 134. Academic Press; 2015:221-240.

16. Flitcroft DI. The Complex Interactions of Retinal, Optical and Environmental Factors in Myopia Aetiology. Prog Retin Eye Res. 2012;31(6):622-660.

17. Jones-Jordan LA, Sinnott LT, Cotter SA, et al. Time Outdoors, Visual Activity, and Myopia Progression in Juvenile-Onset Myopia. Invest Ophthalmol Vis Sci. 2012;53(11):7169-7175.

18. Wolffsohn JS, Calossi A, Cho P, et al. Global Trends in Myopia Management Attitudes and Strategies in Clinical Practice. Cont Lens Anterior Eye. 2016;39(2):106-116.

19. Huang J, Wen D, Wang Q, et al. Efficacy Comparison of 16 Interventions for Myopia Control in Children: A Network Meta-analysis. Ophthalmology. 2016;123(4):697-708.

20. Donovan LA, Sankaridurg P, Ho A, Martinez A, Smith E, Holden BA. Rates of Myopia Progression in Children. Invest Ophthalmol Vis Sci. 2010;51(13):1694-1694.

21. Holden B, Mariotti S, Kocur I, Resnikoff S, He M. The Impact of Myopia and High Myopia. World Health Organization; 2015. http://www.who.int/blindness/causes/MyopiaReportforWeb.pdf.

22. Vasudevan B, Esposito C, Peterson C, Coronado C, Ciuffreda KJ. Human Myopia--Is It Myopigenic?: A Retrospective Analysis of Clinical Refraction Data. J Optom. 2014;7(3):147-152.

23. Gwiazda J, Hyman L, Hussein M, et al. A Randomized Clinical Trial of Progressive Addition Lenses versus Single Vision Lenses on the Progression of Myopia in Children. Invest Ophthalmol Vis Sci. 2003;44(4):1492-1500.

24. Li SM, Kang MT, Wu SS, Meng B. Studies Using Concentric Ring Bifocal and Peripheral Add Multifocal Contact Lenses to Slow Myopia Progression in School-Aged Children: A Meta-analysis. Ophthalmic and. 2017;37(1):51-59.

25. Si J-K, Tang K, Bi H-S, Guo D-D, Guo J-G, Wang X-R. Orthokeratology for Myopia-Control: A Meta-analysis. Optom Vis Sci. 2015;92(3):252-257.

26. Liu YM, Xie P. The Safety of Orthokeratology--A Systematic Review. Eye Contact Lens. 2016;42(1):35-42.

27. Gong Q, Janowski M, Luo M, et al. Efficacy and Adverse Effects of Atropine in Childhood Myopia: A Meta-analysis. JAMA Ophthalmol. 2017;135(6):624-630.

28. Chua SYL, Sabanayagam C, Cheung Y-B, et al. Age of Onset of Myopia Predicts Risk of High Myopia in Later Childhood in Myopic Singapore Children Ophthalmic Physiol Opt. 2016;36(4):388-394.

29. Verkicharla PK, Chia NEH, Saw S-M. What Public Policies Should Be Developed to Cope with the Myopia Epidemic? Optom Vis Sci. 2016;93(9):1055-1057.

30. Phillips T. Taiwan Orders Parents to Limit Children's Time with Electronic Games. The Telegraph. http://www.telegraph.co.uk/news/worldnews/asia/taiwan/11373521/Taiwan-orders-parents-to-limit-childrens-time-with-electronic-games.html. Published January 28, 2015. Accessed January 29, 2018.

31. Council on Communications and Media. Media and Young Minds. American Academy of Pediatrics; 2016:e20162591. doi:10.1542/peds.2016-2591.

32. Gifford P, Gifford KL. The Future of Myopia Control Contact Lenses. Optom Vis Sci. 2016;93(4):336-343.

33. Mani A, Schwartz GW. Circuit Mechanisms of a Retinal Ganglion Cell with Stimulus-Dependent Response Latency and Activation Beyond Its Dendrites. Curr Biol. 2017;27(4):471-482.

34. Gwiazda J, Chandler DL, Cotter SA, et al. Progressive-Addition Lenses versus Single-Vision Lenses for Slowing Progression of Myopia in Children with High Accommodative Lag and Near Esophoria. Invest Ophthalmol Vis Sci. 2011;52(5):2749-2757.

35. Twenge JM. iGen: Why Today's Super-Connected Kids Are Growing Up Less Rebellious, More Tolerant, Less Happy--and Completely Unprepared for Adulthood--and What That Means for the Rest of Us. Simon and Schuster; 2017.

36. Alter A. Irresistible: Why We Can't Stop Checking, Scrolling, Clicking and Watching. Random House; 2017.

37. Schwantes M. Self-Made Billionaire Jack Ma Says You'll Need This 1 Rare Skill to Succeed in the Age of Machines. Inc.com. https://www.inc.com/marcel-schwantes/1-rare-trait-that-actually-trumps-iq-emotional-intelligence-says-billionaire-jack-ma.html. Published October 5, 2017. Accessed January 30, 2018.

38. Ruston D. Screenagers. USA: MyDOC Productions; 2016. https://www.screenagersmovie.com/.

39. What is Captology? Stanford Persuasive Tech Lab. http://captology.stanford.edu/about/what-is-captology.html. Accessed January 30, 2018.

40. Fisk N. "Screen Time" is About More than Setting Limits. The Conversation. http://theconversation.com/screen-time-is-about-more-than-setting-limits-79538. Published 2017. Accessed January 30, 2018.

41. The Eisenhower Matrix: Introduction & 3-Minute Video Tutorial. Eisenhower. http://www.eisenhower.me/eisenhower-matrix/. Accessed January 30, 2018.

42. McChrystal S. Listen, Learn ... Then Lead March 2011. https://www.ted.com/talks/stanley_mcchrystal. Accessed January 30, 2018.

43. Duckworth A. Grit: The Power of Passion and Perseverance. Random House; 2016.

44. Willis JR, Vitale S, Morse L, et al. The Prevalence of Myopic Choroidal Neovascular-ization in the United States: Analysis of the IRIS(®) Data Registry and NHANES. Ophthalmology. 2016;123(8):1771-1782.

45. Teens and Sleep. https://sleepfoundation.org/sleep-topics/teens-and-sleep. Accessed January 30, 2018.

46. Owens J, Adolescent Sleep Working Group, Committee on Adolescence. Insufficient Sleep in Adolescents and Young Adults: An Update on Causes and Consequences. Pediatrics. August 2014:eds.2014-1696.

47. Adolescent Sleep Working Group, Committee on Adolescence, Council on School Health. School Start Times for Adolescents. American Academy of Pediatrics; 2014. http://pediatrics.aappublications.org/content/pediatrics/134/3/642.full.pdf.

48. Klass P. The Science of Adolescent Sleep. https://www.nytimes.com/2017/05/22/well/family/the-science-of-adolescent-sleep.html. Published May 22, 2017. Accessed January 30, 2018.

49. Hagenauer MH, Perryman JI, Lee TM, Carskadon MA. Adolescent Changes in the Homeostatic and Circadian Regulation of Sleep. Dev Neurosci. 2009;31(4):276-284.

50. Hardeland R, Pandi-Perumal SR, Cardinali DP. Melatonin. Int J Biochem Cell Biol. 2006;38(3):313-316.

51. Chellappa SL, Steiner R, Oelhafen P, et al. Adolescent Changes in the Homeostatic and Circadian Regulation of Sleep. J Sleep Res. 2013;22(5):573-580.

52. The Myth of Multitasking. Psychology Today. http://www.psychologytoday.com/blog/creativity-without-borders/201405/the-myth-multitasking. Accessed January 30, 2018.

53. Cui, D., Trier, K., Ribel-Madsen, S. M. Effect of Day Length on Eye Growth, Myopia Progression, and Change of Corneal Power in Myopic Children Ophthalmology. 2013;120(5), 1074-1079.

54. Manuel BD, Lemp MA. Ocular Surface Disorders. JP Medical; 2013.